A Nurse's Story

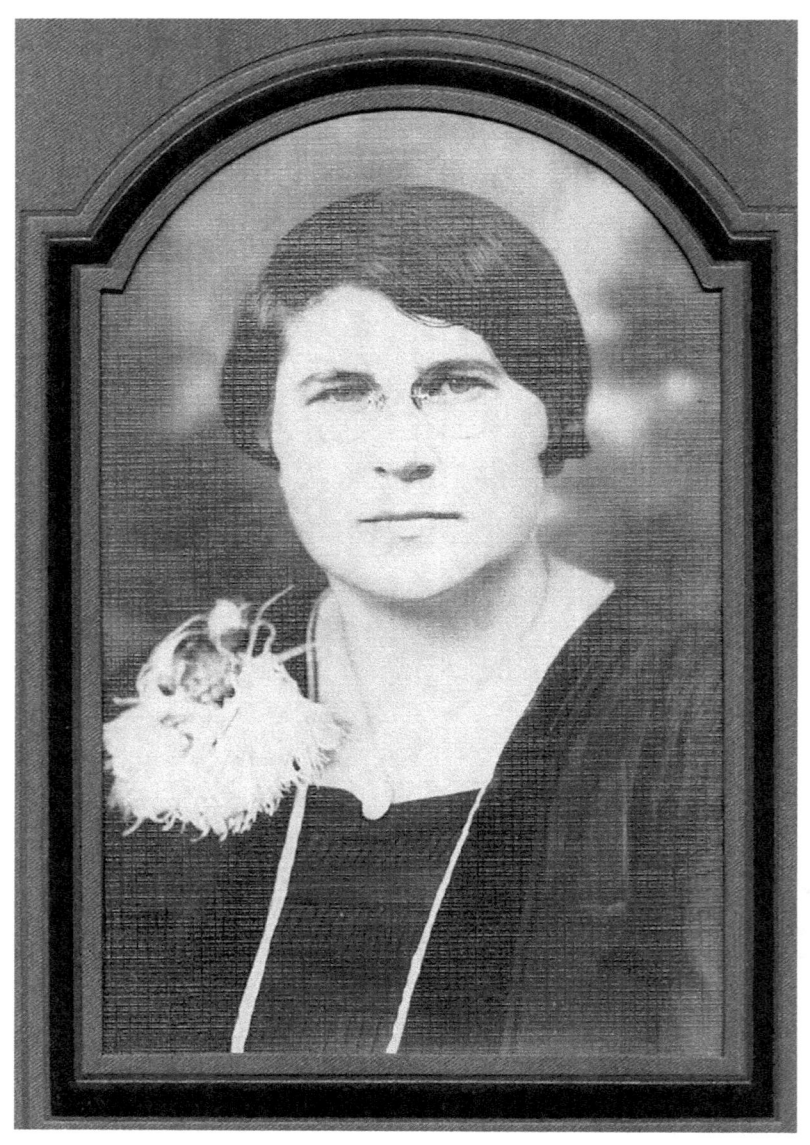
Delia Battles Lewis, 1888-1959

A Nurse's Story:
Medical Missionary in Korea and Siberia, 1915-1920

Delia Battles Lewis

Revised Edition

Edited by
Alison M. Lewis
with John C. Parrish

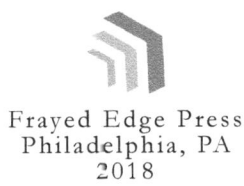

Frayed Edge Press
Philadelphia, PA
2018

Copyright, 2018

Published in 2018 by Frayed Edge Press

Frayed Edge Press
PO Box 13465
Philadelphia, PA 19101

https://frayededgepress.com

This book is printed on acid-free paper

Publisher's Cataloging-in-Publication Data
[Provided by Parlew Associates, LLC]

Names: Lewis, Delia M. (nee Battles), 1888-1959, author. | Lewis, Alison M., 1959- , editor. | Parrish, John C., 1952- , editor. | Goldman, Pamela Lewis, 1932-
Title: A nurse's story : medical missionary in Korea and Siberia, 1915-1920 / Delia Battles Lewis.
Description: Revised edition. | Philadelphia, PA : Frayed Edge Press, 2018. | Summary: Memoir of a nurse who served as a medical missionary in Korea in the early 20th century, as well as in a Red Cross unit on the Eastern Front during World War I.
Identifiers: LCCN 2018933422 | ISBN 9781642510003 (pbk. : alk. paper) | ISBN 9781642510010 (ebook)
Subjects: LCSH: Nurses--Biography. | World War, 1914-1918—Personal narratives. | Korea—Description and travel—1901-1947. | Siberia—Description and travel. | Armenian massacres—1915-1923. | BISAC: BIOGRAPHY & AUTOBIOGRAPHY / Medical.
Classification: LCC RT37.L49 2018| DDC 610.73--dc23
LC record available at https://lccn.loc.gov/2018933422

For all of the descendants...

Contents

List of Illustrations..ix

Foreword - *Pamela Lewis Goldman*......................................xiii

Editor's Introduction - *Alison M. Lewis*..............................xv

Chapter 1 - Early Life and Nurse's Training............................1

Chapter 2 - To Unknown Lands..11

Chapter 3 - Hawaii and Japan..15

Chapter 4 - Korea...27

Chapter 5 - Hospital and Operation...57

Chapter 6 - Dispensary ~ Native Sunday School....................69

Chapter 7 - Korean Religious Life ~
   Visiting in the Country..81

Chapter 8 - Korean School ~ Native Wedding ~
   New Year..97

Chapter 9 - Life in Korea ~ The First World War ~
   Changchun ~ Harbin ~ Refugees.......................107

Chapter 10 - Our Trip West ~ Russian Unrest ~ Thanksgiving in Siberia ~ Typhus Hospital ~ Red Cross Hospital in Omsk...125

Chapter 11 - Our Return Trip across Siberia ~ Independence Movement ~ After the War ~ Severance...........147

**Chapter 12 - New Governor-General ~ Cholera ~
   Ending**..159

Appendix I - Miscellaneous Notes...................................167

Appendix II - Notes on Nursing.......................................175

Appendix III - Obituary..183

**Appendix IV - Typescript of Letter from Miss Shields
   regarding Nursing Textbook**..185

List of Illustrations

Delia Battles Lewis..Frontispiece

Battles Family...3

A Ride in a Rickshaw...17

Japanese Pagoda..23

Interior of a Buddhist Temple..24

A Typical Korean Gentleman...29

Korean Mother and Child...30

Korean Porter with "Jiggy"...33

Korean Hat Maker in Shop...35

A View of Haeju..43

The Norton Memorial Hospital..44

Clinic with Korean Medical Personnel....................................45

Korean Nursing Students..49

Norton Memorial Hospital Staff...59

Women's Ward..61

Preparing for an Operation...65

In the Dispensary..70

"Heathen" Sunday School..77

Piggy-back Sibling Transportation...78

Traditional Korean Janseung Poles 84

In the Countryside: Korean Women and Girl................................91

Korean Village Market................................93

Korean Irrigation System................................95

Korean Bride and Groom................................99

Korean Girls with Younger Siblings................................101

Korea in Winter................................109

The Japan Chapter of the American Red Cross................................111

Russian Horse-Drawn Cart................................118

Russian Hardship................................121

American Red Cross Train Car................................126

The Cathedral at Chita................................128

Life in the Railroad Yard................................132

Soldiers in the Snow................................135

Russian Typhus Hospital................................140

Red Cross Hospital in Omsk................................143

Dressing Warmly for the Siberian Winter................................145

Korean Street Scene................................149

Severance Hospital Nursing Students................................156

Severance Hospital Dispensary................................163

Delia in Traditional Korean Dress................................167

Delia with Haeju Nursing Students................................175

Foreword

Pamela Lewis Goldman

Dear Reader,

When I was a child, one of my greatest pleasures was sitting next to my mother and listening to her retell her adventures as a medical missionary in the faraway land of Korea. Enchanted by the captivating stories and ever so many photographs, I took great delight in being mother's "show and tell." What fun it was to wear the dress of a little Korean girl when she met the demand to be a guest speaker before church and women's groups.

In the years that followed, mother often talked about the need for young women, especially for those who were nurses, to enter the mission field. She felt that if young women knew about the life of a medical missionary, they might be encouraged to do the same. Thus, she began tackling the project of writing her memoirs.

In 1959, at the age of seventy, she unexpectedly passed away leaving an unfinished second draft of her memoirs. Grateful thanks go to her granddaughter, Alison M. Lewis, who took over the enormous task of moving the manuscript forward through a third draft.

Even though there are notes yet to be developed, my niece and I felt that through the internet, mother's hopes to reach young women, as well as nursing women, interested in entering the mission field, will have been achieved.

It is my earnest prayer that those reading *A Nurse's Story* will think so, also.

With love,

Delia M. Lewis's daughter,

Pam

Editor's Introduction
to the original edition

Alison M. Lewis

Delia Battles Lewis was my paternal grandmother, although I never knew her. She died in 1959, a few weeks before I was born. Despite this, my grandmother's presence was very real to me when I was growing up. The brass pagoda, the black stone "idol," and the gilt Orthodox icons in our house were physical evidence of her exotic travels to Japan, China, and Russia that I heard stories about from my parents. I'm sure that Korea was mentioned as well, but it did not stick in my mind in the same way. I remember being told that she had been a nurse and a missionary, and that she had served in "the war"—but I wasn't sure which "war" this was or how all these disparate pieces of her life fit together. I was left with a vague general sense of Grandmother Lewis as a dauntless adventurer, a formidable figure to measure up to. When I took my own trip to China in 1982, I convinced myself to attempt such a long journey by reflecting that, "If Grandmother Lewis could do it, so can I!"

Because there were so many holes in my understanding of Grandmother Lewis' story, I was very excited to learn about the existence of this memoir when I saw my Aunt Pam at a family wedding. I begged her to send a photocopy of the manuscript to me, little knowing the extent of what I was asking. Imagine my surprise and delight when a package arrived containing the original manuscript of over 200 typewritten pages on yellowing paper, along with some typed and handwritten notes. I was fascinated to finally read the story of my Grandmother Lewis' travels, in her own words! The important role of Korea was now clear to me, and the pieces of the larger story started to fall into place.

There were some disappointments as well. The manuscript was written toward the end of my grandmother's life, and since it was a recollection of events that had happened decades earlier, it lacked the detail and emotion that might have been present had she kept a diary or journal during the time of her travels. Also, it was an incomplete draft. There were pages of notes that had not been integrated into the main manuscript, as well as additional notes that had been lost. Her writing was choppy and difficult to follow at times, and because her experience was filtered through the cultural norms of her era, she did not always seem to understand or appreciate the culture she was immersed in.

Overall, however, there are many things of value to be found in this memoir. My friend Bob, who is an historian, pointed out the section in Chapter 9 that describes her encounters with Armenian refugees as particularly significant. This is a difficult part of the memoir to read, recounting as it does some horrific stories of survivors of the Armenian Holocaust. Both the survivors and perpetrators of these acts are no longer living and there is now a movement to deny the reality and the extent of what took place. My grandmother stands as witness, impartially reporting what she saw of the aftermath and what she heard from the mouths of those who experienced firsthand what has been characterized as genocide. In addition to corroborating accounts of those events, her memoir sheds light on other areas of historical interest, including eyewitness accounts of the Eastern Front of World War I, the uprising against Japanese rule in the earliest days of the Korean independence movement, and an account of many aspects of life in pre-modern Korea.

As my Aunt Pam rightly points out in her foreword, this work is also a passionate argument in favor of the value and rewards of the nursing profession, and the work of the medical missionary. My grandmother's concerns for the future of the nursing profession and her desire to present it as an attractive career for young women seem very contemporary, as we continue to hear reports of the on-going nursing shortage. The roles she played in the education of Korean nurses and arranging for the translation of a standard nursing text when none was available in the Korean language, represent professional accomplishments of which she could be proud. The amount of loose notes relating to nursing that were included with the manuscript leads me to believe that it was her intention to include more on this topic in the final version of the memoir, which she was unfortunately unable to complete.

There is something else of interest here as well. In many ways this is indeed the story of the dauntless adventurer that I had imagined my grandmother to be. By all rights, this woman born in the late nineteenth century should have followed in the footsteps of her family and her peers and simply stayed in the small Ohio town where she was born, married, and raised a family. While she did eventually return to that expected path, she first took a whopping detour. She walked out of her family home in Ashtabula, went to the big city of New York to study for a career in nursing, and kept moving all the way back across the continent and around the world. She did something very atypical for women of her generation by traveling great distances to "unknown lands" and placing herself in situations that were unfamiliar, often uncomfortable, and sometimes dangerous. It was an experience that stayed with her for a lifetime and seemed to color everything that came after. Perhaps readers of this memoir may be inspired to take their own first steps out of their comfortable environments and embark upon whatever journey of service and adventure that might await them.

03 03 03

I would like to explain a bit about the process of pulling together this version of the memoir and to thank some of the people who helped make it possible. Foremost is my aunt, Pamela Goldman, who kept the manuscript in her safe-keeping for many decades. She entrusted it to my care and waited patiently through the years that I struggled to find the time and energy to tackle it. She also provided her mother's beloved photo albums of her life in Korea and Siberia. Anyone reading this will surely agree that being able to see some of the people and places described in the memoir adds to its value considerably.

I would also like to acknowledge my friend Robert Helms, whose initial reading and reaction to the manuscript gave me confidence that there was indeed something here worth pursuing. The project would have been slowed considerably, and might not have happened at all, had it not been for the hard work of my good friend, Karen Winner. She took the sometimes difficult-to-read typescript, as well as the typed and handwritten notes, and transcribed them into electronic format so that I could start to work on the text. Thanks also go to Lynn M. Duchez Bycko, Special Collections Associate at Cleveland State University's Michael Schwartz Library. She helpfully located and provided a copy of the *Cleveland Press* newspaper article, quoted extensively at the beginning of Appendix I, which had become garbled in the original manuscript.

Dealing with the manuscript has been a series of "go 'rounds" for me—reading through the text and making corrections, then starting the process again. In the first round, I focused on correcting obvious spelling or grammatical errors, and massaged some of the text into complete sentences. In later rounds, I started to identify place names within the text, many of which had several alternate spellings presented. I did my best to identify the current accepted Western spelling of the location and to use those consistently throughout the memoir. I also did research on some of the people, places, things, and events mentioned in the text, so that I could provide some explanatory information about them in the footnotes. As I learned more about some of the people my grandmother worked with and aspects of the life experiences encountered in the course of her travels, it added greater depth to my understanding of them. I hope my capsule reviews in the footnotes will do the same for other readers.

As has been mentioned, my grandmother was unable to complete the preparation of this memoir before her death, and a number of unintegrated notes or fragments were left behind. In a few cases it was possible to find a logical place within the text to include note material; the rest of the notes have been gathered into the first two appendices—"Miscellaneous Notes," covering material related to Korea, missionary work, the First World War, and other topics; and "Notes on Nursing," covering material related to the profession of nursing. In a third appendix, I have also included a copy of my grandmother's obituary, although not all of the information contained therein is entirely accurate.

I made the choice to maintain my grandmother's chapter divisions and section headings, even when the groupings did not completely make sense to me. I also tried to include some of the most interesting photographs, placing them within the text in close proximity to the description of what is depicted. Unfortunately, there are many wonderful pictures which had to be left out!

In working with the manuscript, I felt a hesitation to change too much of my grandmother's writing. I wanted to retain her "voice" as much as possible, but the prose still felt choppy and difficult to read. It was at this point that the good work of my husband, John Parrish, came to the rescue. He used his excellent editorial eye and greater distance from the subject to apply a different perspective to editing the manuscript. He was able to do what I could not—help the writing flow more easily while still retaining the author's voice. After his treatment, I made yet another "go 'round," making sure that I agreed with the changes and modifying the few with which I did not. In the end I think we reached a satisfactory compromise between staying true to my grandmother's original efforts and creating a more engaging, readable text. For any errors which may be present, I take full responsibility.

Now, more than fifty years after my grandmother's death, I'm happy to make her memoir publicly available. I think it will be of considerable interest to her many descendants—grandchildren, great-grandchildren, and great-great-grandchildren, and generations yet to come. It is also my hope that others outside of our extended family may find something of interest and inspiration here as well.

Philadelphia, 2013

A note on the revised edition

We decided to issue a revised edition of this work in 2018, in order to correct some minor errors, do some additional editing, include some additional photographs, and make print copies of the book available for those who have requested them. The interest in this book, which has been expressed by family members, friends, and strangers alike, has been much appreciated.

I would also like to thank Dr. Sung-Deuk Oak, Associate Professor of Korean Christianity in the Department of Asian Languages and Culture at UCLA, and UCLA's Center for Korean Studies. He has been instrumental in documenting the history of nursing in Korea, including the work of Delia Battles and other medical missionaries.

Alison M. Lewis
Philadelphia, 2018

Chapter 1

EARLY LIFE AND NURSE'S TRAINING

Early Life

My family moved to Cleveland when I was very young. I grew up there and did not return to Ashtabula for many years.

When I was a child, we spent many hours playing in the sand. We would use spoons to dig holes deep down, until we reached our very armpits, trying to see who could dig the deepest hole. Then we would laugh and say we were digging clear through to China. Years later, when I did get to China, I said to myself: "I made it." At that time I did not have even the remotest awareness that I was aiming my life at a goal. Indeed, I was only occasionally aware that there was an outside world.

We always had so much fun as children. In a large family such as ours there were always playmates to be found. We would play marbles or baseball, according to the season. We would jump rope and play hopscotch, and there was a large swing in the elm tree by the house.

We knew where to find beautiful wildflowers: johnny-jump-ups, violets, forget-me-nots, anemones, lilies-of-the-valley, and wintergreens. We knew and loved the local birds; we knew where and how they built their nests, and the color of their eggs. We were fascinated by the young birds with their wide open mouths and would watch the mother birds flying industriously back and forth with rich juicy worms, trying to satisfy their insatiable offspring. We ran races and spent what seemed like eons of time playing "pom pom pull away" and hide and seek. Many a time our mother watched us in amazement and would ask, "Where ever did this tremendous amount of energy come from?"

Winter had its special pleasures: there were angels in the snow and snowmen with eyes of coal, felt hats, and pipes in their mouths. What fun it was to slide downhill! We carried our skates to school with us, so that we could dash to the pond as soon as school was out.

Indoors we played "button, button, who's got the button," pussy in the corner, and musical chairs. When the house vibrated with laughter and we got too noisy with our games, we would hear our father's stern command: "Less noise!" That would compel us to take up quieter games, such as tiddlywinks, dominoes, and cards. We dressed and undressed our dolls, and cut out bushels of paper dolls. Playing dress up in long dresses and high heeled shoes was also great fun.

One of the red letter days of our childhood was our annual family reunion, which we looked forward to and planned for the whole year. There were always new dresses and hair-ribbons for the girls. After our bath the night before, we would place our clean clothes in order on a chair so we could jump right into them in the early morning. There was much excitement getting our large family ready. Mother would give directions and the older children would help the younger ones.

There were baskets to be loaded with picnic food and potato salad to be hurriedly made at the last minute. Father was usually impatient and anxious to get started. We needed to reach the reunion by noon, and it was a long trip by horse and buggy.

The reunions were held at a relative's house, usually on a farm. Long tables with board seats were set up, covered with oil cloth and laden with provisions sufficient for at least a hundred. It was a great day for visiting. There were grandfathers and grandmothers, aunts and uncles, and a host of cousins: first, second, and third. What wonderful dinners there would be! They always started with huge pans of chicken pie being passed, followed by all the other delectable picnic food.

In the early afternoon a business meeting was called for the election of officers. At this meeting we would learn about how our ancestors crossed the Atlantic from England and settled in Connecticut. We also

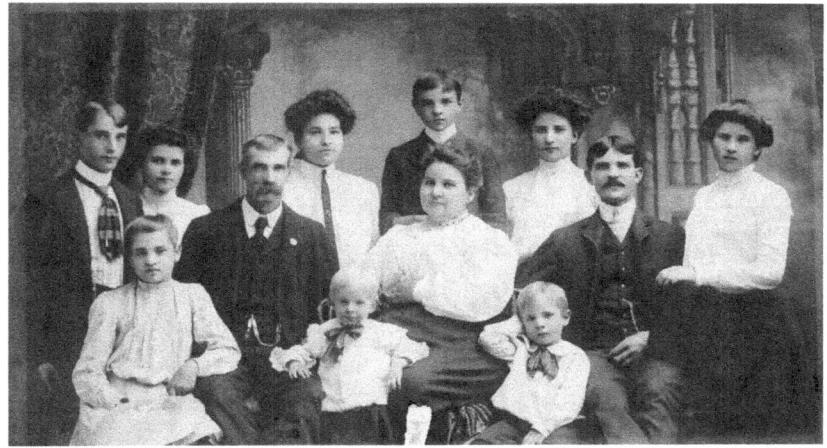

The Battles family. Delia is believed to be the young woman on the far right.

learned about the roles they played in the Revolutionary War and the War of 1812. Following the meeting, the older folks would visit with each other while the younger ones took part in sports and games.

But our childhood was not all play. It was also hard work, for my father was a truck gardener. We were active participants in summer, helping to produce and harvest vegetables and fruit for the Cleveland market. Each child had a special job to perform.

When we were little, visitors to our home would often ask, "What are you going to be when you grow up?" These days, it seems that youngsters can go through college with no idea of what they want to do, but when I was a child, there was never any question in my mind. I always answered, "I want to be a nurse." I do not know just when it was that I developed this notion. It probably came to me when I was quite small, influenced by something I had overheard. It had nothing to do with my knowledge of nurses, for we never had one. There was sickness, of course, and plenty of it, since it took some time for a large family to run through the whole list of contagious diseases. I used to dream of being helpful to people. As I grew older and my knowledge of things increased, the conviction grew in me that nursing was to be my career. I began to shape my plans to enter training.

Maybe it was because of the financial strain of a large family that made me realize early on that I would have to work for whatever I wanted. Dreams would only be fulfilled through my own efforts. Someone reminded me once of an old English saying: "The ball is at your feet," meaning you can stumble over it, you can toss it away, or you can pick it up and run. I decided to pick it up and run.

"Thought will express itself," was an expression I picked up during my high school days. This, and the following two Biblical phrases, had profound meaning for me: "I will hold thee in the hollow of my hand," and "I will guide thee with mine eye." They suggest that life has rough roads and steep climbs. Likewise, at times when cash ran low and I was struggling for my education, I elevated myself with this: "My Father has the cattle in a thousand hills, and he holds the wealth of the world in his hands." With a Father like this, I never had to be envious of anyone!

I never mentioned my mottos to anyone, but stored them up for comfort and strength. I set forth to accomplish my goals with drive and energy, working my way through high school, two years of college, and three years of nursing school. I started out in Ashtabula High School, but returned to Cleveland in my junior year, graduating from East High School. I then had the unforgettable privilege of spending two years at Lake Erie College in Painesville, Ohio, where I came under the guidance of two gracious and illustrious women: Miss Evans, the school president, and Miss Bentley, the dean. Their influence on me left an indelible imprint.

Lake Erie College was noted for its emphasis on athletics, and I joined in wholeheartedly. My game of choice was field hockey, and my position was goal guard. So energetically did I play my part that my teammates called me "Stonewall Battles."

While in college I worked in the dining room, and for two summers I had charge of a fresh air camp for crippled children. The children came out from Cleveland, eight at a time. I worked with them in tents on the grounds of the Rainbow Cottage Hospital in South Euclid, Ohio.

I then spent two years teaching in a one-room country schoolhouse with eight grades in Plymouth Township, Ohio. This provided funds for nursing school and enabled me to repay a small college debt.

Nurse's Training

"Nursing is a hard life," I was warned. However, it was my goal, so I did not waver. I was also shown that a nurse's life represents discipline and training. Three years of study and practice give her skill. Experience gives her judgment. The natural love of mankind makes her willing to fight for life, and gives her joy in bringing comfort and care to the ill.

Through the influence of a friend, I was led to send an application to the Presbyterian Hospital in New York City. My heart pounded as I opened the return letter. I was accepted!

The day I entered Presbyterian Hospital was the fulfillment of a dream. I was joined by girls from various states of the Union, in addition to one from England and several from Canada. They were fine girls: young, energetic, keenly interested, and sincere. When we gathered together that first day in our classroom, we organized the Presbyterian Class of 1915. We felt strange but happy in our plain blue probationary uniforms.

During the first few months we studied our textbooks and spent endless hours struggling with practical demonstrations. We bathed, massaged, bandaged, and spent hours and hours learning to make beds as tight as drums. Our instructors never yielded until we could each make a bed properly. Next we spent two hours a day on the ward, dusting beds and filling water pitchers.

I cleared a major hurdle when I was told to bathe a patient for the first time. I was almost insulted when I was assigned a big, fat, red-faced butcher with a heart condition. Bathe a man, and a repulsive one at that! I was inclined to rebel but by this time obedience had been successfully instilled in me and I had no alternative. I knew the procedure well and carried it out step by step, though I was flustered and dripping with perspiration. It was an ordeal for me, but it finally came to an end. The patient lay there, shining clean in a spotless, tight bed. Then to my surprise, I saw a light steal over his suffering face. He looked up, smiled, and said, "What a wonderful bath." He did not know the rebellion in my heart. My conscience was stricken but I had learned a lesson and met a challenge. Never again have I hesitated to bathe anyone. Through the years my patients have been black, white, yellow, and brown. They have ranged from the most delicate to those who needed a scrubbing brush to get them clean.

Miss Anna C. Maxwell,[1] our superintendent of nurses, was an outstanding personality. Her striking professional dignity filled us with awe, respect, and fear. She ruled as a queen over the whole training school. She had high ideals and a wonderful sense of humor. We stood in mortal dread of being called to her office, but when we were, we marveled at her fairness and understanding.

Our days were full as our training proceeded. We were constantly working with patients and gradually given more and more responsibility. It was a thrill to appear in our blue and white stripes and cap! We were no longer "Probies" and wore our hospital uniforms with pride as we went from the medical to the surgical wards, the emergency room, the children's ward, and then to night duty. In our senior year we were sent with fear and trepidation into the highly organized sanctuary of the operating room. The surgeons at Presbyterian Hospital were internationally known for their skill. Congregating in the dormitory to compare notes, we would pass on bits of gossip and information we had gathered.

---

1. Anna Caroline Maxwell (1851-1929) was the first director of the Presbyterian Hospital's School of Nursing, which was founded in 1892, and later became the Columbia University School of Nursing. Her leadership in nursing education was a major factor in the professionalization of the field. Dubbed "the American Florence Nightingale," Miss Maxwell also organized nurses for military service in the Spanish-American War and World War I, and as a result, was one of the first women given the honor of burial at Arlington National Cemetery.

It was strange to me that people in New York thought my home in Ohio on Lake Erie was "way out west." One day a supervisor asked me why I had come to Presbyterian Hospital. "If I remained in Cleveland I would spend my time off-duty with friends," I told her, "I chose New York because I thought it would be an education to live here." This proved to be true. Not only did I receive excellent training in a school considered to be the best in the country by those of us who attended it, but I gained valuable experience from living in such a cosmopolitan city. There were many interesting places to visit on our time off. We loved the art galleries and museums and visited them frequently. We visited the zoo and parks. Ferry boat rides were fun and we even took a boat trip around Manhattan. We went to shows and occasionally attended symphonies and operas. One thing I did by myself, on my off-duty days, was to visit all the large hospitals in New York City. I even went into their amphitheaters to observe operations.

At the end of our three years of training, we faced our final examinations with apprehension. These consisted of oral and written tests as well as practical demonstrations. We could be asked to do any nursing related task for the practical demonstration. It could be changing a mattress with the patient in the bed, giving a mustard foot bath, making a croup tent for a sick child, or setting up an operating room in a home for an emergency operation.

Our upper classmates had petrified us with horror stories about the doctor who gave the oral exam. "He is one of those doctors," they said, "who loves to confuse the nurse and get her fussed." Discussing it in a jam session one night, one of the girls piped up and said, "Let's just pray we won't have him for our examination." Imagine our surprise when, the night before the examination, we read in the New York evening paper of the death of his mother. We were spared!

The doctor who gave us our examinations was very considerate and behaved like a true friend of nurses. We arrived in the training school office and waited as we were called, one by one, into the Superintendent of Nurses' private office. She remained in the room while the doctor asked the questions. When I was called, every muscle in my body was tense. The first two questions I answered easily. When the third question was asked, Miss Maxwell glanced quickly toward me, then at the doctor. Immediately I sensed that there was something unusual about this question. Was it a trick question or had someone ahead of me been unable to answer it?

The question was, "In what type of a chill is there no elevation of temperature?"

When I answered, "A nervous chill," Miss Maxwell leaned forward with sparkling eyes and looked at the doctor as if to say, "My nurse has answered your question."

The New York State Regents examination came next. We were utterly terrified, even though we knew that no nurse from Presbyterian had ever failed. The examination was difficult. I read through each of the twelve questions and quickly worked out a system. There were twelve questions to be answered. Two of the harder ones I discarded, leaving ten to answer. Since eight would give a passing grade, I concentrated on the eight I felt I knew. With the two I was less sure of I did the best I could. We waited anxiously for the results, and when they arrived weeks later, I had received high enough grades to earn my Registered Nurse degree with honors.

A mail box in the door of Miss Maxwell's office was there for students who wished to write to her. I had one occasion to drop a note in her box. I asked for some work in my senior year, explaining that when I graduated, I planned to go to Korea as a missionary. She willingly gave me the work I asked for, but she could not understand why I wanted to go so far away. In her most majestic way, she waved her hand toward the congested and needy east side of New York City saying, "How can you go away and leave all of this?" I agreed with her that there was great need in the city, but told her I believed greater need existed abroad. Charity begins at home, but it need not end there—the proper sphere of charity is the world. In New York there were many hospitals and clinics. There were special duty nurses, social welfare nurses, and insurance nurses. In one way or another everyone in the city had access to care.

The need for medical help and the opportunity for service were so very great in the mission field. Few nurses were willing to make the sacrifice to leave home and family and go to a foreign country, but I believed that missionary work was most needed, and I wanted to be involved. As an idealistic youth oblivious to risk, I felt compelled to go to an unknown land halfway around the globe. This came as a great surprise to my friends and family.

When I left for Korea as one of the first Presbyterian nurses to go into the mission field, Miss Maxwell sent me off with her best wishes. She freely gave her permission to translate the "Maxwell and Pope" nurses' book[2] when I later wrote and told her of the need for a textbook to train Korean girls as nurses. She also sent a generous gift toward the work of the Alumnae Association. Years later, when I was spending the winter in Washington, D.C., I sought out Miss Maxwell's grave in Arlington Cemetery. Pausing at a little knoll overlooking the Potomac River, I paid silent tribute to one of the true greats of the nursing profession.

---

2. *Practical Nursing: A Textbook for Nurses and a Handbook for All Who Care for the Sick*. By Anna C. Maxwell, superintendent of Presbyterian Hospital School of Nursing, and Amy E. Pope, instructor in Presbyterian Hospital School of Nursing. G. P. Putnam's Sons, New York and London, the Knickerbocker Press, 1907. See the letter from Miss Shields of Severance Hospital regarding the translation of this work, in Appendix IV, page 185.

Chapter 2

TO UNKNOWN LANDS

"Don't you think you are adventurous, to start out alone for a land you do not know and have heard so little about?" I was asked. Service was my aim. But adventure! Yes, I would have that too. At the time—1915—very little was known of Korea. The Western world had taken very little interest in that small country. Perhaps not more than one in a hundred people had even heard of it, or could locate it on a map. While I was there I received letters addressed to Korea Japan, Korea China, and Korea Russia. How different things are today! Every schoolchild in America knows about Korea. Daily papers carry large headlines and magazines are crammed with pictures and articles about the country. The American Army has sent many sons and daughters of family and friends to serve over there.

How glad I was that I was a nurse! Florence Nightingale was my example. She unselfishly devoted her life to the care of the sick and made nursing a respected profession, one upon which doctors have come to depend. I was now being led to broader horizons full of service and adventure through my nursing profession, which I had worked so hard to obtain.

The Methodist Board of Foreign Missions in New York sent me to Korea. I met my traveling companions in San Francisco, who were a missionary family returning to Korea. There were other young missionaries going out for the first time as well who shared my feelings of excitement. Waving good-bye, we tossed colorful streamers from ship to shore. What a thrill it was to board a great ocean liner on our sailing day!

As the gangplank was drawn away our hearts had a sinking feeling, for now we were conscious of the chugging of the motors. Slipping quietly from her mooring, the ship moved out into the harbor where it stopped, remaining all day in San Francisco Bay. We stayed busy that first day by reading our steamer letters, opening our gifts, and settling into our cabins. We explored the ship, arranged our steamer chairs, and enjoyed the magnificent harbor view as we listened to the lapping of the water against the side of the boat. Noon introduced us to the way passengers are fed aboard ship: three delicious full-course meals, a cup of broth in the middle of the morning, and a cup of tea in the middle of the afternoon.

While we were still at the dinner table that evening, our ship steamed out of the harbor and through the Golden Gate. We heard the boom of the breakers against the sea wall. As darkness descended, the wind picked up and the waves lashed. The ship heaved giddily up and then eased giddily down. When we reached the ocean, the ship began to roll. Someone got up and walked quickly out of the dining room. Another followed and then another. A pea green nausea began to creep over me.

"Is this it?" I asked myself. "Has it come to me? I'll not give in; I'll just exercise the power of mind over matter." The ship kept rolling, first one way, then the other. Dishes were crashing to the floor and more and more people were leaving. My appetite was gone, my head was swimming, and I now doubted if it was wise to continue to be brave. I might regret such bravery. Fighting against the roll of the boat, I staggered forward but was helplessly tossed back. Struggling, I finally reached the door and dashed to the deck for fresh air. Standing at the rail were those who had preceded me. Joining them I soon found that the only thing I could keep on my stomach was my hands. Someone passed by and said, "Has the moon come up?" The man who stood next to me groaned and asked, "Does that have to come up too?"

When my friends joined me they asked, "Are you really seasick?" I was too miserable to reply. "The best thing for seasickness is to walk," they said. "Just walk ten times around the deck and you will be all right."

Taking hold of my elbows, two of them walked me around. Once was all I could take, so I pleaded with them to just let me sit down. I dropped into a steamer chair and pulled my robe over me, and there I remained for three days and three nights, too miserable to think. I had little concern for what went on around me; survival was of no interest. It seems we humans were meant to stay on solid ground and not to be tossed about. Our labyrinths[3] let us know we are forcing problems upon them that they were never built to handle. They let us know by making us turn pale, develop a cold sweat, become nauseated, and throw up.

Seasick stories were what well-meaning folks thought they were obligated to stop and tell. All those gay folks who never missed a meal and loved to boast of it took pride in rattling off the whole menu after every meal. I was sure I would never want to eat again as long as I lived. This agony, this utter misery of seasickness, how could one treat it as a joke? Seasickness had one positive benefit: it helped me overcome my subconscious fear of the water. No longer was I afraid that the ship might go down. In my misery I was only afraid that it wouldn't.

My sea legs arrived at the end of three days. I went to my cabin, bathed and changed, and joined my fellow passengers for a delightful voyage. There was a gleam of hope now, and we were floating along under happier stars. Walking the deck freely, my feeling of adventure was released and flooded my being. The further from home I went the more I sensed the feeling of being a part of the universe, no longer bound by routine nor fear of the water. I looked at the gorgeous canopy of the heavens, the constantly shifting, fleecy clouds floating past, and I was thrilled at their beauty. It was a marvelous experience seeing sky and water meet to form a circled horizon. The night sky, too, was fascinating. It changed from light blue to dark blue and then when the twilight was gone, the moon and stars came out. From the blue of the heavens to the blue of the water, the moon spread a sparkling path of silver before us.

---

3. Here the author is using the term "labyrinth" in its anatomical sense: "A group of complex interconnecting anatomical cavities," most likely the gastro-intestinal system.

The stars and planets above took on new importance as they shone down on us. I felt that I was among friends. The same heavenly bodies had always been there in the heavens. They had fascinated me as I had picked them out, one by one, so many times as a child: there was the North Star, the Big Dipper, Venus, and Mars. Out here, as we headed into the southern waters, they seemed so close. It was as if they knew we needed something familiar to comfort us in the middle of the Pacific Ocean, and so they came down a little closer. Here, surrounded by the beauty of the heavens, I was overwhelmed by the utter insignificance of man in the vast expanse of the universe.

Several days and several hundred miles out, the sea was no longer a stranger. I no longer felt I had left security behind and was facing danger ahead. These were wonderful days, gliding along on a smooth sea, with God in His heaven above.

There was a great deal of diversion aboard ship. There were sports and games, concerts, and Sunday services. We loved to watch the water, searching for whales and flying fish.

After we had sailed for two weeks, our journey was half over and flocks of gulls were seen flying overhead. Circling, they appeared to be looking for a spot to rest. Surely land must be near! Soon we observed a dull gray line upon the horizon, and Honolulu appeared in the distance. I had a tremendous urge to cry out, "Land, land!" as Columbus and his sailors must have done when they came to America.

The water was calm as we drifted into the harbor.

Chapter 3

Hawaii and Japan

Hawaii

Hawaii: the crossroads of the Pacific. The fabulous islands!

As the ship glided into harbor our attention was first attracted to a group of young native boys swimming and diving about the ship. Passengers tossed coins into the water and watched the boys splash and scramble until one lucky one would come up smiling. He would show the coin, store it away in his cheek, and be ready to dive again. With bulging cheeks, the boys kept up this sport as long as we stood on the deck tossing coins.

How wonderful it was to place our feet once again upon good old Mother Earth! We spent an entire day in this tropical fairyland, a unique and intriguing storybook world. Fragrant flowers were in abundance amidst rich and luxuriant foliage. Remarking on the frequent rains someone explained: "In Honolulu, one gives directions like this, 'Go up the street for two showers then turn to the left.'" They call these rains "liquid sunshine."

A beautiful city, Honolulu is situated at the base of two volcanic peaks, each with an elevation of at least 3,000 feet. A motor trip to the top of the one called Pali gave us a magnificent view. In one direction we could look out over the sea and the surf on Waikiki Beach. In the other were great fertile fields of pineapple. The people we met were obliging and courteous; they appeared to be friendly, kind, and likable. We longed to know more about their fascinating islands but our time was limited.

Thrilled with our day of sightseeing, we dashed back to the ship that evening at sailing time and soon found ourselves out to sea once more. Churning through the water day after day we learned to enjoy the restful and easy life aboard ship. We did not find this difficult because it was so tranquil and unconstrained. I had often dreamed of sailing across the ocean and now that my dream had become reality, the reality seemed like a dream.

One day we were knifing smoothly through calm water when I suddenly became aware of a new sound—a fog horn. We had encountered fog for the first time and the horn's mournful rolls could be heard over the grinding of the engines. The anxiety this aroused in me was somewhat out of proportion to the danger.

"How long will the fog last?"

"Does it cover the entire ocean?"

"Are there other ships close by?"

It was like a bad nightmare, like finding oneself drawn to the edge of a high crevasse with an unknown drop ahead. Shut in by fog, one had the impression of standing still in space, covered and surrounded, with no lighted path toward which one might turn, the firmament embracing the world. The haunting sounds issued by the fog horn every five minutes did not help to dispel our fear, even though we were told that half our fear was baseless and the other half discreditable. This was before the days of radar. We hoped no other ships were in the fog near us, but if our ship was traveling its usual speed, it was covering considerable distance in the five minutes between horns. Left now to the mercy of God, we worried until the fog horn ceased, and when it did, we accepted the silence with blissful relief. Slipping peacefully through calm waters, we counted the days to our next port, Yokohama.

Japan

Japan was in the midst of a gala holiday when our ship glided up to the dock at Yokohama. A coronation was being celebrated. Brightly colored banners, Japanese lanterns, and huge paper fishes hung from

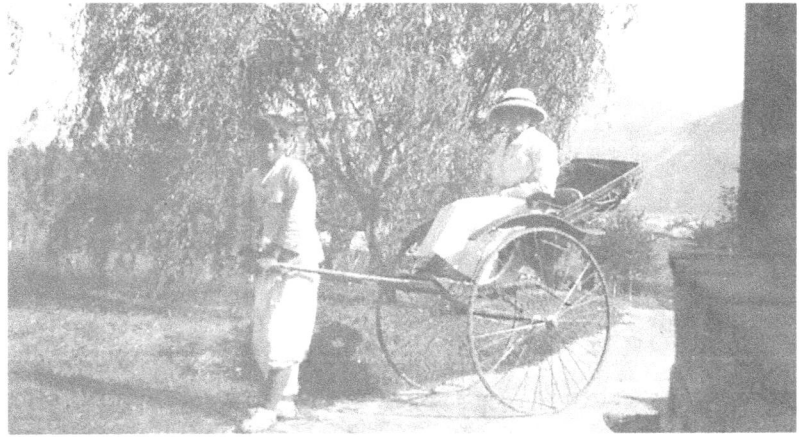

A ride in a rickshaw

the buildings. It was a great festive occasion. How fortunate for us! Because of the coronation our ship remained at Yokohama for three days instead of one. To take advantage of this wonderful opportunity, a party was quickly formed to go sightseeing.

Once we were ashore, an unfamiliar sound attracted our attention: the clack, clack of the wooden shoes worn by the Japanese. Their white stockings resembled mittens except that the separate place usually reserved for the thumb went to the big toe instead. A strap coming up from the shoe fit between the big toe and the next, holding the shoe in place and helping the wearer to scuff along.

Anxious rickshaw men awaited passengers, so into one of these high, two-wheeled, man-drawn baby buggies we stepped. Our rickshaw man was unique. He was dressed in what appeared to be a pair of men's long winter underwear, with a blue belt and loin cloth. He also had a piece of cloth tied about his brow which he took off from time to time to mop his face. Many a time I had wondered what people in other countries thought of our newspaper and magazine advertisements, especially the ones where people are all dressed up in their underclothes, standing there smiling. Papers, magazines, and even the Montgomery Ward catalog had reached this country; here was a man who had evidently dressed himself up in American style.

The rickshaw, I was told, was invented by a Chinese missionary whose wife was an invalid. He converted a baby buggy into a carriage so that his wife could be drawn about. The vehicle, now much improved by rubber-tired wheels, has become one of the chief methods of transportation in the Orient. Fear of falling backward lessened my enjoyment of the ride. The Japanese, on the other hand, rode along with great dignity. We were soon in the hustle and bustle of the busy narrow streets, gaining our first impressions of this fascinating country.

Men and older women were dressed in somber colors, while young women and children wore gorgeous, brightly-colored kimonos. Ladies were girdled with a beautiful and expensive sash called an obi. Many native men appeared in Western clothes. Crowds of people in rickshaws, carts drawn by bullocks, street cars, the occasional automobile, and people on foot jammed the narrow streets. Japanese-made bicycles were everywhere. They darted in and out, this way and that, perilously complicating our progress. Once we turned into the business section, the streets became wider.

Zigzagging our way through terrible traffic, we went first to the house of the president of Japan's largest steamship company. Aboard ship, the passengers had all received an invitation to tea. Arriving at a magnificent palatial building, our rickshaw men dropped the shafts of their vehicles and out we stepped. The building had an artistic, eastern design and was surrounded by a large, beautiful lawn with many shrubs and trees. We were ushered up a wide carpeted stair and into a fairyland of the most gorgeous rooms.

The rooms were larger than those of ordinary houses and had no windows, but were walled with sliding screens. They were finished in especially fine woods that were polished, not painted. The ceilings, divided into panels by lacquered strips, were exquisitely designed. Expensive silks, painted with Japanese scenes and intricate patterns, hung on the walls. In contrast to all of this oriental beauty were modern electric light fixtures. The exquisite art on display throughout the rooms made me feel as if I was in a museum.

In the large reception room, we were served ceremonial tea with all the dignity of the tradition. I was too overwhelmed to even note that part of the ceremony. I do remember lovely young Japanese women dressed in colorful kimonos bowing as they served us handle-less cups of delicious tea. We found it most refreshing.

For the Japanese, the drinking of a cup of tea has special meaning. Japanese etiquette requires an atmosphere reflecting purity of thought, peacefulness, reverence, and relaxation. To complete the essentials of a perfect ceremony, the best tea must be used, served in the finest cups, and the tea must be served with proper manners. Since the United States is Japan's biggest tea market and has been known to import more than a million dollars' worth in a year, isn't it too bad that our hyperactive, ulcer-suffering country hasn't learned to quiet down and take time to observe the ceremonial tea service?

Visiting this magnificent home was an unforgettable experience.

Traveling in Japan

How interesting it was to travel about Japan! Off the main highways the countryside was so picturesque. Narrow paths led into cool, shaded, beautifully landscaped spots. Rippling streams with waterfalls were crossed by artistic rustic bridges, and there were pretty little tea houses where tea and cakes were served.

Japanese landscape gardening is considered by many to be ahead of the rest of the world. It has been developed as an art form for hundreds of years. A preparatory study is made of every detail; the effect of the trees, shrubs, water, and stone are carefully planned. Usually working within a small space, the finished effect will look much larger than it actually is, producing a feeling of spaciousness.

The Japanese have perfected the art of dwarfing trees. From ancient times they have developed techniques for growing them in pots, with limbs that are gnarled and twisted into picturesque shapes. When one sees a gnarly, foot high pine rooted in the crack of a rock in a Japanese garden, it is hard to believe that it might be a hundred years old or more. An ancestral tree may have received devoted care throughout the lifetime of the father and grandfather. Stones of different shapes and sizes are also used to great effect, although flowers and their colors do not play as prominent a part in landscaping as one might think. Nonetheless, the Japanese are noted for creating skillful flower arrangements, which they use in homes for decoration. Much attention is paid to the symbolism of the flower. They pay more attention to line than color, and bend and snip until the twigs and stems make an artistic effect.

We boarded a train and soon found ourselves in Tokyo, the capital. Tokyo is a curious city, an interesting mixture of east and west. We saw lovely eastern goods in beautiful shops, while nearby were large Western-influenced buildings featuring goods brought in from all parts of the world. Signs over the doors were in English as well as Japanese.

Tokyo is situated on beautiful Tokyo Bay and occupies a greater area than any other city of comparable population in the world, covering approximately one hundred square miles. One- and two-story homes are the norm because of earthquakes that frequent the region, although some of the more modern builders have put up buildings seven and eight floors high using steel and concrete. This practice has seemed daring to many and the buildings have been viewed with suspicion, but so far they have withstood the shocks of earthquakes.

Tokyo is the political center of Japan and is a busy, bustling city. It is the seat of government, and is gradually growing in world importance. On one sightseeing trip we saw the large business section, the railroad station, bridges, and street after street of homes that were walled and windowed with paper. We also saw the Imperial Palace with its spacious grounds surrounded by thick walls and a moat.

In the eyes of the Japanese people, the Emperor is divine. He is always given the sincerest respect, courtesy, and esteem. When he passes by in the street, all traffic stops and the people stand with bowed heads. To look down on the Emperor from an elevation is considered most insulting. Devotion like this was difficult for us to understand. We were told this story: One day, while he was making a visit to a Yokohama railway station, the Emperor's private car was switched to one side in the yard. At a certain time the car was to be brought back and made ready. Upon returning, the Emperor had to wait two minutes for his car. The station master was so humiliated and filled with remorse to have caused his Emperor such an inconvenience that he committed hara-kiri.

After the doors of Japan were opened by Commodore Perry, the Japanese advanced rapidly toward a modern civilization. They are excellent imitators and absorbed ideas of colonization from England, military practices from Germany, and educational systems from America. Because they found Chinese men to be honest, they entrusted them to head the banks. Promising young men and women were sent to foreign countries for advanced study, with the government paying all expenses. These people returned from abroad with new ideas to promote within their own country. So eager were they to copy that I saw English perfumes and soaps, even Ivory soap, on their shelves. Not only did they manufacture these things themselves, but they used the same type of paper and copied the trademarks.

Their capability for imitation and urge for progress showed in many ways. I was told a story aboard ship that illustrated this. When the Japanese first accepted modern Western civilization, they had England build all their ships and used English officers to man them. As the country advanced, however, they wanted to begin building their own ships. A Japanese company ordered a ship from a London shipyard and asked for plans and specifications to study. Then they copied the plans in minute detail and returned them, stating that they had decided against placing the order. They built a ship from the plans but when they tried to launch it, it nearly toppled over. To protect their plans, the English company had purposely included errors, but by removing a deck and adding ballast, the Japanese were finally able to successfully launch the ship. It was on this same ship that I crossed the Pacific Ocean. I also heard the story of a Japanese man who bought an English cotton mill. Time passed and there was no repeat order; the English firm never heard from him again. Years later, when the firm sent a representative to Japan, he was given the address and told to look up the man. Arriving at the address he found a fully functioning factory! The cotton mill had been taken apart, minutely copied, and many duplicates were made. Today, Japan is among the world's leaders at manufacturing cotton.

In Tokyo we visited Mitsukoshi, which is Japan's largest department store. As we entered, we noticed that people were leaving their shoes and going into the store in stocking feet. What were we to do? We paused in wonder, but our embarrassment was soon relieved; an attendant offered to slip soft cloth slippers, held snug with rubber elastic, over our shoes. This enabled us to walk over the beautiful floor mats without fear of getting them dirty or marring the fiber with our heavy shoes. The store was large and beautifully decorated. Even the goods for sale added to an artistic effect. There were bright spring kimonos, gaily colored oil paper umbrellas, lacquerware, shoes, jewelry, and pictures. They seemed to have everything!

When night arrived, we found a Japanese inn where we could spend the night. At the entrance we removed and checked our shoes. Walking across the highly polished veranda, we entered our matted room. The walls and partitions were of paper. These sliding screens were in sections and moved back and forth in grooves. They could open to the outdoors, or several rooms could be made into one large room.

On the clean, rice straw mats that covered the floor, we would sit as well as sleep. Without tables, chairs, or beds our rooms were quite bare. The only decoration was a small alcove. The alcove is the focal center of the room, and a scroll is usually hanging in the recess. Underneath it might be found an object of art, such as a bronze vase, an exquisite piece of pottery, or a flower arrangement. In our American clothes we found it very difficult and miserable trying to sit on the floor. The Japanese are so very graceful; they put their knees together and descend like a folding knife to sit on their heels. We hunched around, sat tailor fashion, or extended our feet out in front of us: all postures that the Japanese would consider most disgraceful!

That night we slept in Japanese fashion. Coming in and bowing low, the little maid gave us two thick quilts that we were to sleep between without sheets, and a small hard pillow. So tired were

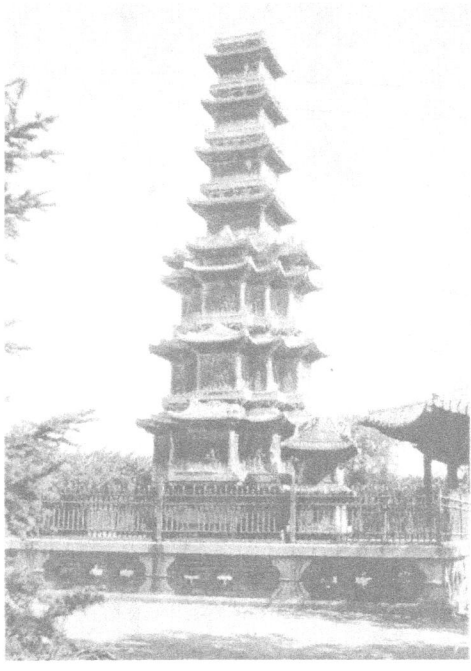

Japanese pagoda

we from our hard day of travel and sightseeing that we soon fell asleep, despite our unusual bed on the floor. Refreshed by our sleep, we were ready the next morning for our trip to Nikko.

Nikko

We were intrigued by Nikko, which is considered to be one of the most sacred spots in Japan. Nikko means "sunny splendor," and it is rich in beauty, legend, and lore. We were told that it is so beautiful that the Japanese have a saying: "See Nikko and die." There is nothing more worthwhile to see.

It was our good fortune to visit in the fall and see Nikko dressed in gorgeous autumn colors. Trees cloaked in rich reds contrasted with fragrant green pines, and the colorful shrines were wonderfully impressive. Nikko is where the most perfect collection of shrines in Japan can be

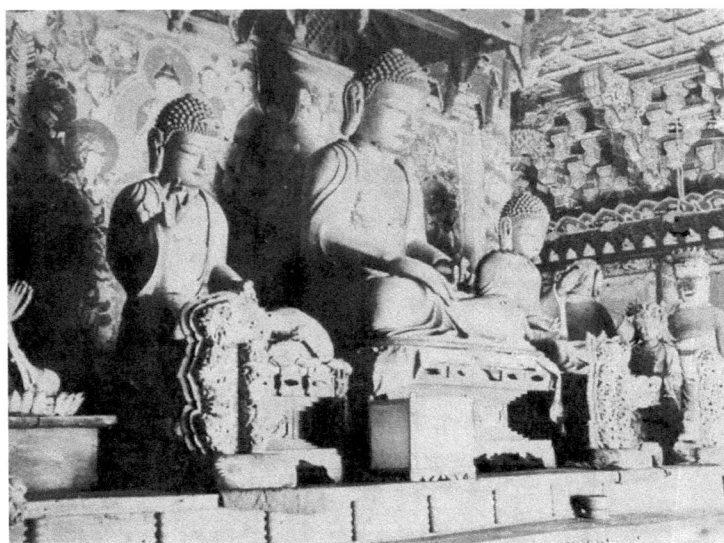
Interior of a Buddhist temple

found. These shrines reflect the religious beliefs of Japan, the two principle ones being Shinto and Buddhism. Elaborate gates called torii mark the terraces leading up to the shrines on a hillside. Pagodas and temples can be found in addition to the shrines. These are in wooded settings, often accompanied by fountains and waterfalls. The shrines are typically one-story buildings of oriental architecture, rich in color. Red predominates, but some are blue, yellow, green, gold, and brass, with Chinese tiled roofs made from green copper. Marvelously wrought carvings decorate the buildings. There are golden doors and beautifully decorated ceilings, with red and gilt used in abundance.

Inside the temples were statues of many gods. Some, like Buddha, had a placid expression, and some were ugly. At Buddhist shrines a pleasant tinkling could be heard as breezes swung wind bells back and forth.

Mount Fuji

Fuji, the sacred mountain of Japan, is a dormant, snow-capped volcano, reportedly with a huge crater at the top. Shining in the bright sun and appearing to rise out of the sea, it slopes gently upward for 12,000 feet. Standing alone, it is a majestic monarch with its white cap piercing the sky. It is not surprising that such an artistic people as the Japanese worship this beautiful mountain.

Love for Mt. Fuji is ingrained in the Japanese people. Many shrines are built on its slopes, and it is considered a mandatory pilgrimage destination. All Japanese feel the need to visit the summit at least once during their lifetime. The mountain has an important symbolic role in the religion, art, and literature of the people. I found its image on many daily objects: fans, tea cups, screens, pottery, paintings, and exquisite embroideries.

It is the unfortunate traveler who passes across the lower part of Japan on a rainy or overcast day and misses this magnificent picture. It was my good fortune to cross the region three times: once by train and twice by ship on the Inland Sea. In each instance I was blessed with a beautiful clear day that allowed me to fully appreciate the beauty of this glorious mountain.

Leaving

The engines were already chugging as we boarded ship, and we soon sailed out of Yokohama Harbor. Sailing through the Inland Sea, our next stop was Kobe. Then, with a sense of regret, we left beautiful Japan, the land of the Rising Sun, with her intensely patriotic and strongly nationalistic people.

Chapter 4

KOREA

Korea

There is always a fascination when entering a new country. The journey across the strait from Shimonoseki, Japan to Busan, Korea took a few hours in a small boat. I was happy to step ashore, for this was to be my adopted home for the next five years. Throughout Asia, Korea is known by its ancient name Cho-sen which means "Land of the Morning Calm," a reference to the characteristically clear and beautiful mornings which occur during much of the year.

Picturesque Japan was left behind. This was a different land and my eyes were distracted by every new and strange sight. There were white-robed men with peculiar hats and an odd rack on their backs, often bearing enormous loads. The women, also dressed in white, would stand erect with a jar or basket on their heads or walk along quietly in their straw shoes. Children wearing gay, brightly-colored clothes followed closely behind their mothers. Oxcarts, rickshaws, and pedestrians moved solemnly down narrow dirt streets between low shops and houses. Hills could be seen in the distance that, except for an occasional green patch, had been denuded by fuel gatherers.

What of the first impressions? The dust, the open sewers emitting contaminated air, the flies, the soiled white garments, and the running noses of the children were evident, but I could discern within the heart of each person I saw a human soul, reaching out for light, understanding, and the chance to grow and develop their latent possibilities. Obliterating all thoughts of prejudice and allowing only kindness and compassion to fill my heart, I resolved that nothing would daunt me. I rededicated my life to service, and there arose in my heart a love for these kindly people. I had come all this way to find the King's Highway in Korea and now I was grateful to be here. There opened before me a fascinating experience, filled with adventure and enough excitement to provide a lifetime of memories.

My traveling companions, missionaries returning from furlough, watched me closely. They wanted to catch my reaction and first impressions, in hopes of reliving the thrill they once had on entering the country for the first time.

At Busan we boarded a modern, well-equipped, American-made train, and arrived ten hours later in the capital city, Seoul. High officials and foreigners patronized the five first-class cars. I was now a foreigner, a stranger in a strange land. The well-to-do of the country rode in the second-class cars. The third-class car was far from comfortable and had wooden benches for seats, which were occupied by people of lesser means. The first railroad built in Korea was a short line linking Seoul to Incheon. An American company built the line from Busan to Seoul. Then, during the Russo-Japanese War, Japan got permission to transport troops across Korea after agreeing to complete the railroad to the Yalu River.

Seoul is a most interesting place, with a quaint, eastern atmosphere. All Koreans hope to get there at some point in their lifetime. Some streets in Seoul are wide, while others are extremely narrow. The native homes are stone and mud-walled; roofs are tiled or thatched with rice-straw. The government built many of the large modern buildings, including the post-office, bank, hotel, and schoolhouses. Others were built by missionaries, including hospitals, churches, schools, colleges, the YWCA, and the publishing house of the British and American Bible Society. A small streetcar runs from the East Gate to the West Gate of the city, with a branch in the center running between the South Gate and the railroad station.

Although everything moves along in a leisurely manner, there is much activity in the streets. Cows with huge loads of wood on their backs provide a means for supplying the fuel for cooking rice, the principle food. Oxen hitched to crude carts transport large loads, and bicycles are seen in great numbers. Rickshaws dart about, pulled by runners carrying single passengers. If a party is traveling together, the rickshaw men run in a line, each close upon the other. Added to this scene are great numbers of pedestrians, dressed primarily in unique native costumes, interspersed with the occasional man in Western clothes. The native costumes for men consist of white balloon-like trousers tied at the ankle with a cerise-colored ribbon. There was usually a cotton blouse covered by a full, loose coat of cotton or silk. These coats were tied with a single bow of material on the left side. They wore stockings made of white cotton and their shoes were straw, wood, or some combination in slipper style. Their tall, black horsehair hats looked like flower pots turned upside down and were kept on by black string tied underneath the chin. The hats impart a dignified air. The hair, which could be seen through the loosely-woven hat, was drawn into a top-knot on top of the head.

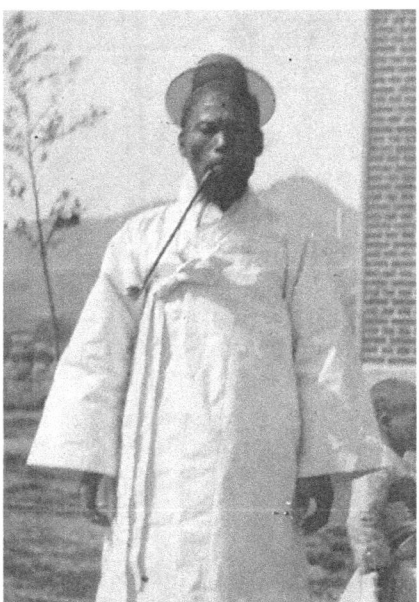

A typical Korean gentleman

There are customs in the East which seem to be the opposite of those in the West. White, for example, is the color of mourning, and because several years might be spent in mourning for a king, and a certain length of time for each member of a family, the people spend much of their time in white. White has eventually grown into a national color. Women spend many hours washing and ironing to keep their families spotlessly clean.

Korean women are modest and retiring. They live a quiet and secluded life, their dignity unknown to the world. They receive satisfaction from the esteem of their husbands and pleasure in the happiness of their family. The women wear long, full skirts held fast by bands tied just below the armpits. Just above the skirt bands is a very short waist. Both skirt and waist are tied in a single bow at the left side, with the streamers hanging. Underneath the full skirt, a pair of large balloon-like trousers are worn which cover the length of the body from chest to ankles. Silk, cotton, or homespun linen are the primary fabrics used for their clothing. They dress mostly in white, although young women wear

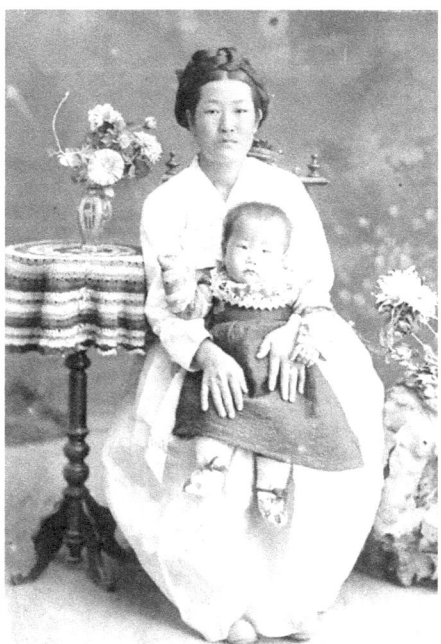

Korean mother and child

pale blue. A brightly-colored winter hat is worn in some sections of the country. In others, a turban is worn which is made of folded white cloth, somewhat in a Roman fashion. Most of the women, however, wear no head covering at all. Their black, oiled hair is drawn straight back with a coil made at the back of the neck through which they put one hair pin, usually a small bar of silver or wood.

Children wear garments similar to those of their parents, but of gay bright colors. Each mother makes her son a jacket, the sleeves fashioned from one inch strips of brightly colored fabrics laid side by side. It reminded us of Joseph and his "coat of many colors." We found many things in Korea that reminded us of the Old Testament.

Lost

I got lost in Seoul on my second day there. Assuring my friends that I could cross the city alone, I started out for the Mission Hospital. Because of my poor sense of direction, however, I transferred to the streetcar for the West Gate instead of the East Gate. When I reached the end of the line, I looked around expectantly but could see no hospital. Confused, bewildered, perplexed, and panic-stricken, I looked about and could only see a few laborers working on the road. My skill with the Korean language was restricted to a few expressions my friends had taught me while we were on our ship, such as: "Good morning," "How are you," "Doctor" and "What is this?" One friend told me, "Never become discouraged about the difficulty of learning the language. Never waste a minute crying over it, just keep at it. Keep asking, 'What is this?' and countless nouns will be revealed." Unfortunately, "What is this?" would not help me now, and neither would "How do you do?"

Approaching the workmen, I looked toward the hill where the hospital should be and said "Doctor." After looking at each other they pointed in another direction. Fate, destiny, or divine will intervened just then. A missionary who lived near the West Gate observed the situation and came to my rescue, pointing me in the right direction. When I finally reached the East Gate at the other end of the trolley line, I looked up at the hill and there was my hospital. Infuriated at myself, I vowed to learn my way around the city. The very next day, believing that I could get the lay of the land better by walking, I set out to do just that.

Seoul is situated in a valley surrounded by mountains. As I walked along I noted the street car tracks set in the middle of the fairly wide business street. Slow moving bullock carts passed along and here and there were cows with brushwood stacked to great heights on their backs. Delivered to the homes, this wood was used in native fireplaces for cooking and heat. Rickshaws were in evidence, pulled along by their jogging attendants and I even saw an occasional pack pony.

Pedestrians walked quietly along attending to their individual business, each representing a different stage of society. The typical Korean man is of medium height with a well-shaped head. He has a gaunt, almost expressionless face, placid, faintly slanted black eyes, and a finely chiseled nose. His skin is yellow, his hair is coal black. Sitting or standing, he appears relaxed and casual. He gives an impression of kindness, generosity, wisdom, and endless patience. He moves slowly, as if there is no reason for haste, walking with a very erect posture and a poised, dignified air. Many of the old men have straggly beards with hairs so sparse one could almost count them. Over the centuries Korean men have become almost beardless. All are dressed in white. Laborers can be identified by their tanned, leathery skin and soiled garments. They are the exception to the rule, since men in spotless white can be seen everywhere.

One figure in particular stands out: the yong-bang. A nobleman, he is usually dressed in white or pale blue silk. In his black horsehair hat, he walks along with a nonchalant, swinging gait, literally strutting along the street. As a scholar, he is widely admired and looked up to, and he often has a following. He lets his little fingernails grow long to show that he never does anything as undignified as manual labor. Rigid etiquette forbids him to take any but official or tutorial jobs. When these are unavailable, he must sponge off more fortunate relatives or risk losing his dignity.

I saw fewer women than men on the street, and these were mostly of a lower class. Women are quite secluded. Members of the better classes will usually be seen only in rickshaws or in a partly covered chair, mounted on two poles and carried on the shoulders of four men. One woman I saw had a jar on her head and a baby strapped to her back. Underneath her short waist were exposed breasts. Shocked and embarrassed, I said to myself: "I am glad I am alone on this trip." While in Korea I saw many such women and later discovered that this was a culturally accepted aspect of motherhood. At that time there were no bottle-fed babies in Korea, so wet nurses were common. I even saw old grandmothers hushing up fretful babies by offering their withered flabby breasts as human pacifiers.

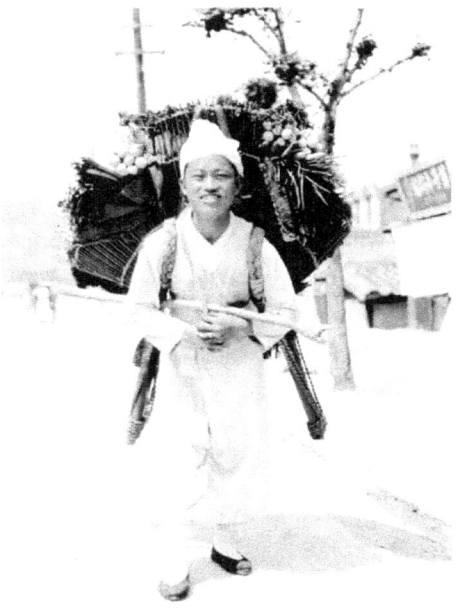

A hardworking Korean porter with his "jiggy"

Here and there, the good-natured porters known as "jiggy men" trudged along, carrying tremendous loads on their backs. Prior to the introduction of trains, human muscles were the chief method for transporting goods. The "jiggy" is a crude but clever device with a frame comprised of two forked sticks, or peeled branches of trees, the length about that of the head and trunk of a man. They are laced and tied together and supported by the man's back. Loops of rope go over the shoulders and underneath the arms, and the two protruding forks form a shelf on which the load is placed and tied. The men rest their jiggy on the ground as they secure their load, propping it up with a forked stick. Then they kneel down with their back to it, thrust their arms through the two padded loops at the side of the frame, hunch it up on their backs and walk right off, often with a two or three hundred pound load. I once heard of a missionary having his piano carried this way on a man's back. I was personally carried for some distance on the back of one of them after becoming exhausted on a mountain climbing trip. A missionary doctor who tried to open an abscess on the back of one of these men had a great deal of difficulty cutting through his tough skin, even with the sharpest of scalpels.

Water carriers with two pails slung on ropes hanging from a yoke across their shoulders can be seen splashing along using pails made from Standard Oil tin cans. The locals use these tin cans in many ways. I was surprised to learn that large American corporations such as Standard Oil and Singer sewing machines were already present in this far-off land.

Turning from the busy, dusty street, my attention was drawn to the small shops on either side. The buildings flanking the street are single-story structures with curved tile roofing and the wide part of the building open to the street. These local shops open out onto the sidewalk during the day and are boarded up at night. One merchant squatted tailor fashion in the middle of his shop with all his goods no more than an arm's length away. They were in small piles on the floor, on low shelves, or hanging from the walls. His goods were inexpensive and not particularly interesting, but were adequate for the simple needs of the people. There were short lengths of cotton cloth, skeins of cotton thread, straw shoes, wooden combs, tobacco pipes and pouches, dried fish and dried seaweed, writing paper, small blocks of black ink, and brushes for writing. The people who stopped to make a purchase were making payment with a greenish bronze coin that had a square hole in the middle. Each coin may have been worth a tenth of a cent or less.

In another, more prosperous shop, the placid merchant's commodities included stacks of narrow, coarse, native homespun cotton cloth, horsehair hats, pottery, candlesticks, combs, pipes and tobacco, spittoons, horn-rimmed glasses, dried persimmons, dyed candy, kerosene lamps, and hand mirrors. Another, much more interesting shop caught my eye because it contained real Korean crafts. There were several sizes of brass food bowls, brass chop sticks, and spoons. There were brass incense burners in graceful shapes and patterns, black lacquered pieces inlaid with mother-of-pearl, and beautiful embroidered textiles patterned with silk and gold thread. Interesting and well-made bureaus and marriage chests were also for sale. Some were of solid chestnut while others were veneered with maple or peach, bossed, shaped, hinged with brass, and ornamented with great brass padlocks. These uniquely Korean chests are handsome and distinctly decorative.

Merchants are often seen squatting on the floor of their open shops or passing their time by whittling. One had several sizes of wooden combs, wooden hair pins, and wooden shop stickers for sale. Another

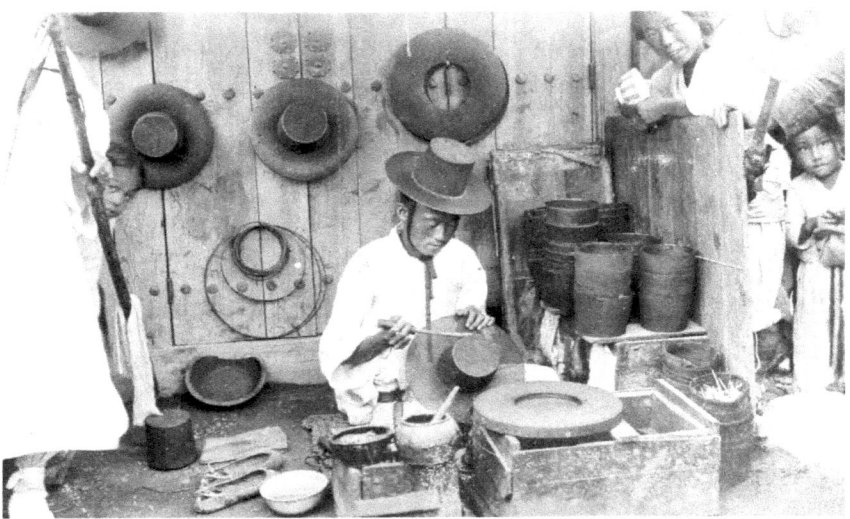

A Korean hatmaker in his shop

shop contained many shapes and sizes of pots and jars for sale. The potter turns his wheel with his feet. As the wheel turns, the clay begins to take form. He works with his hands and a few basic tools: a wooden spatula, a trowel, a curved stick, and some rags. I saw Korean potters making beautiful clay jars and bowls with a lustrous glaze. There are examples of Korean ceramics, some made as early as 900 AD, which can be found in museums around the world.

Pottery is made in all shapes and sizes and is used to store grain and food supplies, as well as to carry laundry, usually perched on a head, back and forth to the stream. Some pots are nearly as tall as a man. These are used to store and preserve their native pickle, called kimchi, which is made from chunks of long white turnip and slices of Chinese cabbage, heavily salted and sometimes seasoned with red pepper. Shrimp is added to one variety.

The jars are buried in the ground up to the brim, then covered and left to season. Most households will prepare a supply in the fall that will last for many months. Kimchi is eaten daily and is an important part of the Korean diet. A standard meal usually consists of a large bowl of rice, a large bowl of kimchi, a small side dish of fish—substituted occasionally by beef or chicken—and a bowl of rice water or seaweed soup. When we learned of the seaweed soup, which is rich in iodine, we understood why goiters were rare in Korea. Honey water tinted pink, with nuts floating on top, is a native delicacy that is sometimes served as well.

Koreans eat with chopsticks and a shallow spoon made from brass, or occasionally, from silver. Wooden chop sticks are universally used, and a traditional and precise etiquette is observed at meals.

As worthwhile and informative as this trip was proving, I felt I had learned my lesson for the day so I retraced my steps. I walked along in the strange crowd alone and unnoticed, without attracting the slightest curiosity. Even if I had generated any interest, the stoical Koreans would have been unlikely to show any outward sign.

Things Korean

The ancient kingdom of Korea was called Ko-li. Outside of the country today it is known as Korea, while the natives call it Cho-sen. It is an elongated peninsula lying off the southeast corner of Manchuria and is bound on the east by the Sea of Japan, on the south by the Chosen channel,[4] and on the west by the Yellow Sea. Six hundred miles long from north to south, one hundred thirty-five miles wide from east to west, it is approximately the size of New York and Pennsylvania combined, composed of an area of over eighty-four thousand square miles.

Mountain ranges run the length of the land. The eastern division is a narrow strip of fertile land between the mountains and the Sea of Japan. The western part of the country has many rugged foothills and mountains. These mountains and hills are beautiful and picturesque, with small towns and villages nestled on hillsides and valleys. Homes are built with mud and stone walls and roofing of thatched rice straw. From a distance they look like so many mushroom patches.

Approximately eighty percent of the population farms the land; the slopes and valleys are irrigated and well-suited to agriculture. Fishing, mining, and small business enterprises are also important occupations.

There are presently[5] about twenty-two million people in Korea. They are proud of the fact that their history dates back over four thousand years and smile indulgently when we tell them how old our country is. We are just too young to be taken seriously! In the early centuries of its history Korea was the highway on which civilization marched from China to Japan, bringing important advances in art, science, and industry.

---

4. Now more commonly referred to as the Cheju Strait or the Jeju Strait.

5. This manuscript was probably written in the mid- to late-1950s and this population estimate dates from that time. 2017 population estimates are approximately 51 million for the Republic of Korea (South Korea), and approximately 25.5 million for the Democratic People's Republic of Korea (North Korea).

Japanese records indicate that they also gained various skills from the Koreans, including architecture, art, landscape gardening, and pottery (including the famous Satsuma ware), as well as how to cultivate the silk worm and weave cloth. Books were printed in Korea as early as 1234 AD, and the spinning wheel was first used in 1370 AD. In 1446 AD, King Sejong devised the Korean phonetic alphabet, a system so simple that one may learn to pronounce Korean words in a few days.

Korea has long been referred to as "The Hermit Nation," but few people know the reason why. From 1592 to 1598, the Japanese devastated much of the Korean peninsula in an effort to conquer China. The Koreans finally repulsed the invaders when Admiral Yi Sun-sin invented the first iron clad ship called the "Tortoise Boat." Their ship sank the Japanese fleet, which was attempting to transport reinforcements to Korea. Remembering this terrible invasion, Koreans allowed no foreigners to enter their territory for the next three hundred years.

In 1882, after Commodore Perry's arrival opened up Japan to the West, Korea signed a treaty of peace, amity, commerce, and navigation with the United States. Two years later, the first American missionary landed. At first Korea did not welcome foreigners. At that time there were sign posts on the streets that said, "If you meet a foreigner kill him. If you let him go you are a traitor to your country."

Once they began to see the material advantages of the West, however, some Koreans had second thoughts. They began to pick up new ideas which were the invisible cargo that came along with the strange new material goods. However, some of the more alert Koreans saw a great door sliding open and worried about their country. If they stepped out through this door, they would enter a vast new world, the world of modern civilization, forever leaving behind their own world which had known little change for thousands of years. While many tried to cling to the old world they had always known, the more venturesome felt the irresistible pull of this new world being brought to them by the West. Once having seen this vision of the outer world, the urge prevailed. They longed to know more.

Korea's isolation and lack of development made it vulnerable to more advanced nations. Situated between Japan and China, it was often invaded from one side or the other, serving as the battlefield upon which the two powers fought. When Japan went to war with Russia in 1904, its leaders sought Korean permission to transport troops across the country. Permission was granted but when the war was over, the Japanese did not go home as promised. Instead, they stayed and occupied the country. The Japanese assassinated Korea's queen,[6] which aroused intense anti-Japanese sentiment among the people. The Korean king[7] had always been friendly with Western Christian missionaries and received comfort from them during the troubled time of the Japanese occupation. Some of these missionaries told of delivering food to the king in a locked box. This was all he dared to eat, so fearful was he of being poisoned.

Japan made Korea a protectorate in 1910, incorporating it into the Japanese Empire. The Japanese military government was in power in Korea when I arrived in 1915. Soldiers were to be seen everywhere, policing the country. Teachers in the government elementary schools went about among the little children with swords clanging at their sides.

Away from the commercial sections of Korean cities, the people live in a labyrinth of alleys so narrow that a man can barely pass a bull with its load of wood. The houses are closely huddled together and are all single-story, since custom forbids two-story houses. The alleys are not only narrow but also crooked, rocky, and muddy, with open sewers running along the sides. Many people I know would have found it to be a most desolate and miserable place. I found fascination in everything I saw, however, and never allowed myself to become discouraged or depressed.

---

6. Empress Myeongseong (1851-1895), also known as Queen Min, wife of King Gojong. She is said to have been killed by sword-wielding assassins sent by the Japanese military.

7. King Gojong (1852-1919), also known as Emperor Gwangmu, first emperor of the Korean Empire. He was forced by the Japanese to abdicate in 1907, at which time the Empire was briefly ruled by his son.

The backs of Korean houses face the street, so one sees a stone and mud wall with a small door. Many of the houses have a court around which the rooms are built. All rooms are eight feet by eight feet in size. The women of the house live in the inner or separate rooms. The outer room nearest the gateway by the door is used by the male members of the family.

The method for warming the houses is peculiar to Korea. The floor is paved with stones and plastered over with clay. Flues run the length of the house and serve as both a chimney and a furnace. The kitchen stands at one end of the house with a large iron kettle cemented in an arch over the fireplace. The same fire that prepares the food heats the house. Dried pine twigs, grass, and split wood are used as fuel. The heat-laden smoke passes through the flues and out a low chimney on the opposite end of the house, heating the floors on its way out. Radiant heating has been used by Koreans for centuries.

The floors are covered with a tough native oil paper, kept clean thanks to the custom of removing shoes when entering the house. On the warm floors of these rooms people sit cross-legged in tailor fashion. Rooms are adapted for sleep at night by rolling out two narrow cotton blankets, one to lie on and one for cover. A small hard pillow is used to support the head. Many people will simply loosen the bands of their garments and sleep with their clothes on. Often, several people will sleep in a room.

Koreans have been slow to adapt to modern civilization. They prefer a simple, primitive life, retaining from their ancient civilization many admirable qualities. For example, they are gentle, deliberate, and polite, regarding anger as the most inexcusable of sins. They are mild, calm, quiet, and even tempered. They are humble, not overbearing or oppressive, and are rarely hasty in judgment. They dwell more in the past than in the future. They observe filial piety and bestow honor, obedience, respect, and reverence upon their elders. A Korean child would never think of calling his father "the old man."

The longer I lived among the Korean people, the more they intrigued me. I discovered that, despite their unique racial and national characteristics, they were human beings not so different from us. Sometimes there is too much division in the human family. One race feels superior or one nation feels superior. But nations and races are all made of people, and the Koreans are people. They see, they hear, they feel. Their hunger is satisfied by food. They hurt the same way, and when they are ill, they seek healing. They have homes, wives, husbands, and children whom they cherish. They labor to feed their young and they fight to protect their families. They too dream and care, hope and pray, laugh and wonder. People are the things they say; people are faces and the expressions on them. People are personalities. Personalities represent types. I was surprised to find in Korea similar personality types to those we have at home. I learned that people are people, regardless of their color or where they live.

Traveling North

In the middle of the railroad station as the crowd surged around me, I stopped and blurted to the doctor who had come to conduct me on the last lap of my journey: "I don't think I want to go." Startled, the doctor realized he had a problem. Here at last was the much needed nurse, all the way from America, and now she didn't want to go north to the hospital.

"Why?" he asked.

Things were still pretty primitive in this country, and an older missionary in Seoul, to prepare me, had told me what to expect on the journey to Haeju. One traveled by train from Seoul to Inchun, and there boarded a small coastal steamer. This was a twenty-four-hour trip that started at night, and there was only one cabin. All passengers used the one cabin and slept on the floor.

"I just don't want to do anything out here I wouldn't do at home," I stammered.

He must have done some quick thinking, for he responded, "I sized you up to be a person who could face any situation you met."

I went on.

The water seemed so dark at night; there was only a lantern here and there on the dock for illumination. With fumbling steps I got into a sampan, which rowed us out to the steamer. In the majesty stillness of the night, with some misgivings and a bit terrified, I listened to the rhythmic dipping of the paddles and the lapping of the water on the sides of the boat. "Have no fear," reassured the doctor as we boarded the steamer. "There is no danger; this boat makes a daily run up and down the coast."

Our sailing time was governed by the tide. I learned then that Incheon has the second highest tide in the world. With the clang of a bell and a call of "all aboard," we felt the ship slowly pull away from the dock. Soon the dark strip of water between the boat and shore grew wider and wider and the lights on the shore grew dimmer.

As we headed for the open sea I tingled with the realization that I was headed, not for the jumping off place, but for what was to be an adventure into the great unknown. I was excited and impatient to face the uncertainty, and thrilled at the anticipation of new experiences and discoveries.

We found the cabin as described. Since it was quite late, we prepared for the night in true Oriental style. Placing a folded steamer rug on the matted floor in a corner close to the wall, I lay down with my clothes on and drew a blanket over me. I was the only woman in the cabin and slept that night with the missionary doctor, a Chinese man, two Korean men, and three Japanese. Dozing lightly, I desperately clutched my pocketbook and prayed for the dawn.

All the next day, we sat on deck and enjoyed the beautiful coastal view as our steamer chugged north through the Yellow Sea along the picturesque western shore of Korea. At one point we passed a whole fleet of Korean fishing boats, each manned with naked men. Although Korea was a fine old civilization, certain aspects seemed quite primitive.

Toward evening we arrived at our destination harbor and found a group of Korean Christians and missionaries with eager faces bringing greetings of welcome to the new nurse. Most of the Koreans walked the three miles to the harbor and back again. We rode to the city in rickshaws.

Haeju[8]

In a beautiful valley surrounded by mountains and hills lay the picturesque city of Haeju. This was my destination; I had come a great distance. I stood now firmly on the ground that was literally rock beneath my feet. Firm enough, I trusted and hoped, so that my hand would not tremble as I stretched it forth to bring comfort and enlightenment to the people of Korea. Such was my prayer. A contemplation of God's work developed in my heart, combined with a love for the people and a generous concern for the good of mankind. With youthful exuberance, I prayed that I would be able to maintain the standards of my ideals—to

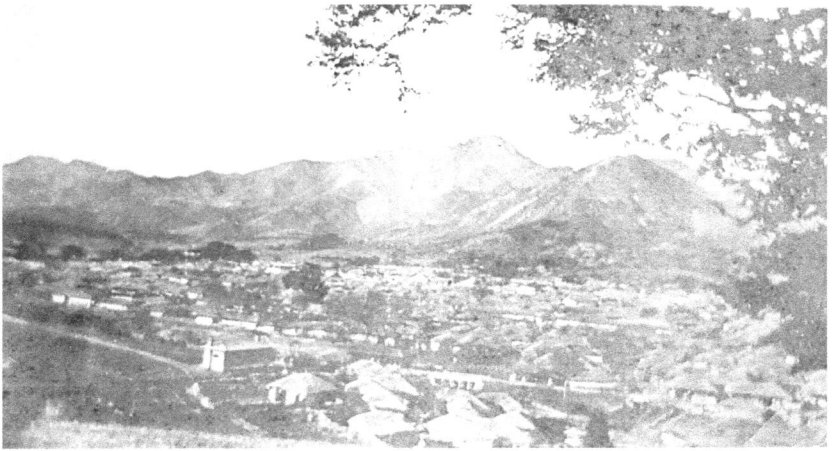

A view of Haeju

the extent that my capacities and surroundings would permit—through dedication to a life of service. I prayed also that when difficulties, hardships, and trials came—as they surely would in due course—that they would strengthen me and help me grow in character and grace. It may seem strange to some that we should be happy here, but truly, what could be more worthwhile or rewarding than to meet the needs of thousands

---

8. Haeju now has a population of over 241,000 and is the capital of South Hwanghae Province in North Korea.

of people untouched by Western medicine? The help we could give was so meaningful. Through our contact with the people at the level of their daily lives, we could share in their problems and provide them with sympathy expressed through the service we gave. This human contact can open a new way of thinking, a new way of life to the people, and to a nurse this is a most rewarding experience. Nothing could be more wonderful than being a nurse right here, where the need was so great.

The mission hospital seemed to dominate the city even though it was on the outskirts. It stood on the side of a hill and was easily accessible. A modern red brick building only two stories tall, it nonetheless towered above the native homes. The Norton Memorial Hospital was the fulfillment of a dream for Dr. Arthur Norton, who was its founder and director. He dedicated the facility to his mother, and through it, was able to achieve his wish to bring modern medicine and care to the people of the region. Further up the hill and quite apart from the native cottages stood a group of missionary homes that seemed like part of the hill. In the middle of this compound flowed a bubbling spring that supplied all of the fresh water for the missionary homes and hospital.

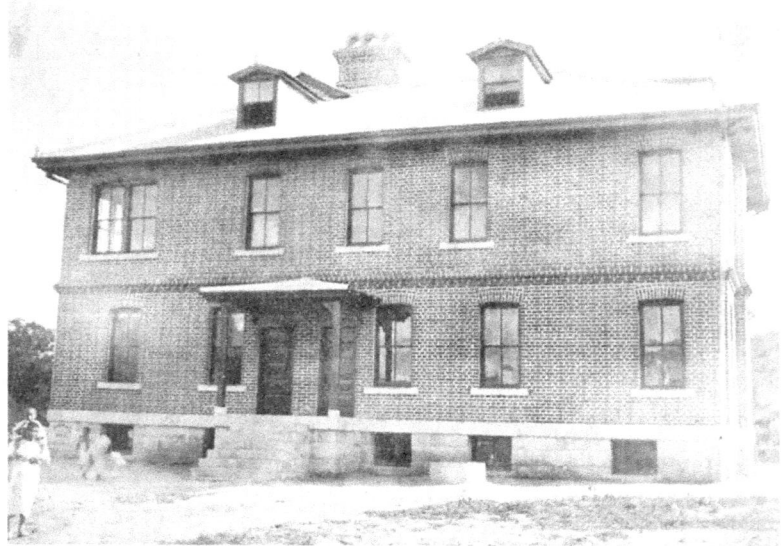

The Norton Memorial Hospital in Haeju

I felt so fortunate to find this brand new hospital waiting where I could begin my missionary work! The moment that the door was opened I was struck by the typical, undeniable smell of a hospital: ether, iodine, alcohol, and something boiling. I was immediately at home. The hospital had a ward for men, a ward for women, a couple of private rooms, two offices, and an operating room. It also had a drug room, a dispensary, and a waiting room. The doctor had a personally trained assistant and there was a pharmacist. With the assistance of four nurses-in-training, we could care for fifteen to eighteen patients a day in the hospital and about eight hundred patients a month in the clinic. We had to make the most of the few supplies we had; linens were limited and our dressings and bandages were often washed and re-sterilized.

I saw a Korean nurse working with a patient; she came forward to meet me. How I longed to know her intimately. She smiled so sweetly, squeezed my hand, and clutched my elbow. I knew there was a bond between us. I had an odd feeling that we were in the same world, and as nurses we understood the same things—we recognized a need. There was an urge within us to serve which could bridge the barriers of race,

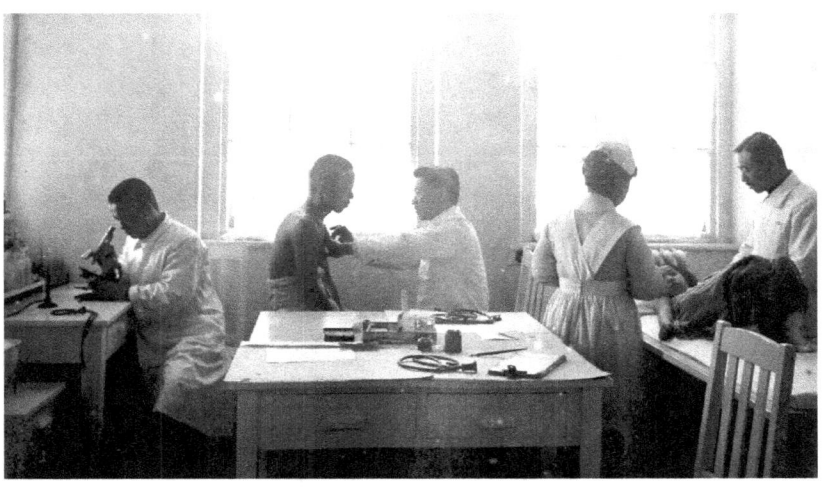

Clinic with Korean medical personnel

color, and language and allow an understanding to grow between the hearts of kindred souls. I felt a love in my very being for this girl which expanded over time into a feeling of love for all the Korean people.

The mission hospital had only twenty beds, but represented a real luxury for the people. The Koreans called it the "Salvation Hospital" because they knew that here they would not only have their wounds dressed and their sufferings relieved, but they would learn of the Great Physician as well. Many of our patients went from the hospital into the church. As medical missionaries we did not have a cloistered and academic existence—just the opposite. We had to keep our sleeves rolled up, for there was always plenty to do in the hospital.

I was happy to be there and anxious to get started in the work at once, but I found I had a language barrier. Difficulty with understanding the language beset all new arrivals and it became my problem too. At that time there was no language school for new missionaries. There are many things nurses can do without knowing the language, however, and since I was right there in the hospital and seeing the work that needed to be done, it was tempting to keep busy and let the language problem slide. I had a private instructor, a young Korean student who was learning English. Since I may have been a better teacher than he, I thought sometimes he learned more of English than I did of Korean. In time, I developed a passing knowledge of the language, but never became really fluent. It would have been useful to have been provided a period of dedicated language study on arrival, to become better oriented before starting to work.

Transplanted into Korea, I found an environment there which was entirely different from anything I had previously known. In fact, many things were just the opposite from what I was accustomed to. For example, in Korea the family name comes first. They read from the back to the front of the book and from the right to the left. Men are always first. They are served food first and women eat what is left. The appreciation of this food is indicated by the amount of noise made while eating. When a husband and wife walk down the street, the wife walks demurely about six feet behind, carrying a baby on her back and their luggage on her head. Men wear their hats in the house but leave their shoes outside when entering. They sit and sleep on the floor. The chimney runs underneath the house. Waving the hand, which to us means "good-bye," to them means "come on." When you meet someone for the first time, they always ask how old you are. They also inquire how much you pay for things. Few have watches, so they arise to the new day at the first or second cock's crow. A day's work runs from sunrise to sunset. You never ask a woman if she is married, you ask if she has gone to live in her mother-in-law's house. We were training two young men as nurses since it would be culturally inappropriate to let female nurses take care of the male patients. Separate rooms were maintained even in homes, and in the churches there was a partition down the middle, with men on one side and women on the other.

To the Korean, who is always slow and deliberate, time has little meaning. "After a while" seems to be their motto. They move slowly and are never in a hurry. If a thing is not accomplished today, any time will do. Although they have half a dozen words that mean "hurry," calling out one or all of them would not cause a Korean to quicken his step. In the hospital, however, time is important. One must fight for time to save a life, time to stop a hemorrhage, time for a drug to take effect.

Walking down the narrow, stony paths to the main street of Haeju one day, I tried to analyze what I had learned about the Koreans so far. I had observed their lives and customs and studied their private and public ways of doing things. If what I learned seemed strange and unusual to me, I wondered what they thought of us. We had come to sing songs of Zion in a strange land. Did we not feel a sense of pride? Were we not confident that we had come to this land to live a life of glorious service and self-sacrifice?

Suddenly there was a commotion behind me, which made me turn. There, to my surprise, was a Pied Piper mob of small children, following me and crying out "Foreign devil, foreign devil." I took note of the tousled hair, dirty faces, soiled garments, and wooden shoes of my small followers. I was immediately dashed from my sophisticated consciousness and made to feel quite puny. My elation at feeling indispensable was definitely flattened.

We all know the difference between giving and receiving. As the giver, one soon learns that it is easier to be generous than grateful. Doing for others expands you, builds you up, and stiffens your spine. But as the receiver, one has to either do something to earn the gift or demonstrate gratitude, or the gift might break your personality. The Bible tells us it is more blessed to give than to receive.

Koreans must look in wonder at Westerners who hurry, worry, and always try to make those around them move faster. How strange these white people are; it is hard to understand them. The missionary soon realizes that he too has a lesson to learn about time. He finds that if he wants to understand the Korean people, he needs to slow down and take his time. Otherwise, he is unable to help them.

Training Korean Nurses

Establishing a training school in the northern interior of Korea presented real difficulties at this time. Attracting young women to the hospital for training meant bringing them out of seclusion. Also, the high standards for nursing that we knew at home had not yet been established here. Many Koreans looked upon nursing as the lowest kind of labor; taking care of the sick was viewed with disdain. Many contradictions existed among the Korean people between their needs and their beliefs. This was illustrated by the case of a very sick baby that was brought to us. The family obviously loved the child or they wouldn't have chosen to go to a foreign hospital. "Why didn't you bathe the baby?" I asked, as I noted the dirty little face wrapped in a soiled blanket. The mother looked at me with surprise and said, "Is it possible to bathe a sick child?"

Another obstacle made the search for suitable nursing candidates difficult: the lack of Korean girls with a reasonable foundational education. Before the arrival of missionaries in Korea, girls were not allowed to go to school. A woman wasn't expected to learn such things as were taught there. It was enough that she know how to wash, iron, cook, sew, and

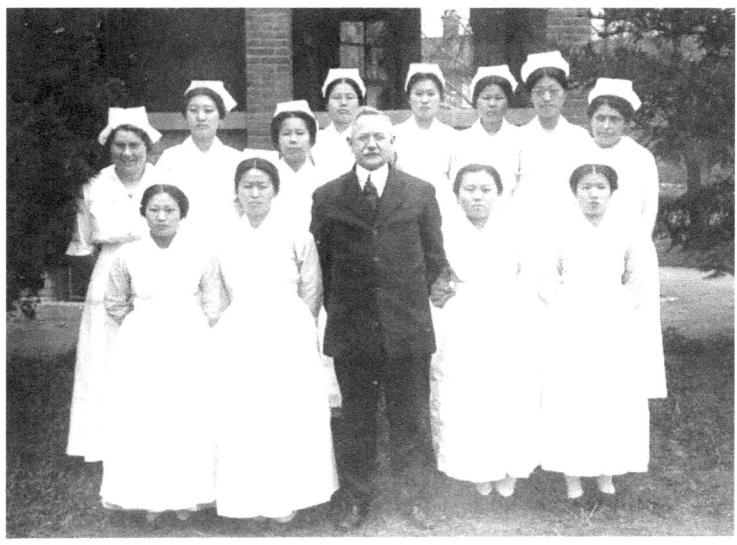

Korean nursing students with Delia Battles (far left) and Dr. Norton

take care of her babies. Fortunately, a missionary grade school for girls had already been established in Haeju. With some of the graduates of this school and a few widows with limited education, we began to build up a class for nurses training.

Our candidates had no idea of nursing when they arrived, and my attempt to tell them how everything must be done was difficult for them to comprehend. As a foreigner, I was strange and whatever I said was strange. They had never heard such things before and they often did not get my point. Why should just five drops of medicine be given, no more and no less? Why not give a very sick patient anything he wants to eat? Why does it make any difference if a patient is given the treatment tomorrow instead of today?

Eastern pride was inexplicable to us and we found one of the hardest things to teach the girls was the dignity of labor. For example, there was the simple task of dusting. I told them many times that dusting was a nurse's duty, necessary for the direct protection and welfare of the patients. Nonetheless, it was difficult for them to see the necessity of it. One nurse was heard to say that she was ashamed to go before patients and dust, because it was servant's work. This remark was made by a girl who came from the poorest of poor country homes. But not all of the girls were like this one.

The mission training school had many problems. We drew our students from untidy homes with ignorant parents. These girls had, at most, the opportunity of only a few years' study at the mission school. As a result, we could not start their training at the same point that training schools would typically start in the United States. They lacked the foundation of knowledge, culture, and poise that help a home nurse to take up her professional career. In addition to helping them acquire the specialized knowledge and skill required for their duties and responsibilities as nurses, we had to instruct them in matters of personal cleanliness, honesty, exactness, punctuality, orderliness, and purity of thought. Fortunately, they were friendly and hospitable, with a strong desire for knowledge. They were also optimistic and extremely patient, with a keen eye for detail and the ability to readily imitate. Because of these qualities, the young nurses under our tutelage were soon able to do many things. In order that they might look their part, we dressed them in nursing uniforms. A uniform has a distinctive association with the nursing profession and inspires confidence in patients. It is invaluable to the wearer and helps to remind the nurse that no task is too humble to perform when the need of the patient requires it.

In the laboratory, we introduced students to the microscope where they could view the tiny, unseen world of Korea. Here were the beautiful and deadly shapes responsible for leprosy, tuberculosis, malaria, cholera, and typhoid, as well as the eggs of worms and other intestinal parasites. They had never heard of Lister's germs or the theory of antisepsis. They knew nothing of asepsis, pasteurization, or sterilization. General hygiene was unfamiliar. They looked on placidly, making no outward sign of surprise or emotion, but by watching the germs dash madly about, they were able to see for themselves the need for cleanliness, asepsis, and sterilization.

In order to run the mission hospital properly, it was essential to train native nurses. It would be impossible to supply enough American nurses to staff the hospital, and the expense would be prohibitive. Native nurses were also necessary to quell the natural fears of the people, who were suspicious of foreigners. Had they not all heard the tale that the foreigners stole little babies and gouged out their eyes to make medicine? It was understandably easier to have confidence in a nurse who could understand the Korean point of view. She could listen patiently to a man who described his trouble by explaining that the old Korean doctor had stabbed a red hot needle into the abscess on his arm to let the disease devil out, whereas we would have reacted with disgust. She could quietly explain that the modern doctor had a better method. She could also provide reassurance by supplying the names of his friends who had been helped at the hospital. She would soon have him willing to have the abscess opened.

Our training school established that Korean girls, given an opportunity, could be trained to be excellent nurses. They surprised us with their patience and inherent ability to imitate; they quickly caught on. We marveled all the more when we saw their progress with sterilization. How were they able to transition from homes with no running water to a spotless modern hospital? This backward northern city was blazing a trail for nursing, although similar schools had been established in large cities like Seoul and Pyongyang.

Dr. Norton was cooperative in all aspects of the training school and aided in the instruction of the nursing students. Our trainees were beginning to be in demand, even those who had not yet completed their training. We sent one to another city to take care of a typhoid patient under the supervision of a mission doctor. Several others had opportunities to care for missionaries who were ill. In this way we were able to help out in missionaries' homes where there was illness, and this gave the trainees experience in Western homes, caring for Western patients.

The "cona-one-john" (general-of-nurses), was the title the Koreans gave me. My position certainly required many roles: instructor, supervisor, and head nurse. I gave anesthetics and sometimes assisted at operations. I also gave the important treatments, tracked the charts, and occasionally stayed the night with an extremely sick patient.

At this time there were no textbooks, nor was there any literature in Korean on the topic of nursing. The lessons I wrote out were translated into Korean and passed out to the class, which I taught through an interpreter. Later, I obtained permission from the authors and publisher to have the Maxwell and Pope book of nursing[9] translated into Korean. This came out in mimeograph form and proved a great help in our training schools.

My work was not without its discouragements; there were many obstacles to overcome. Sanitation was primitive. Modern medicine was almost unknown. There were not even words into which medical terms could be translated. The patient's fears had to be overcome before their confidence could be gained. As foreigners, we nurses and doctors must have seemed very odd; we looked and acted like people, but we were so white! We had blue eyes, something absolutely unknown in a nation of dark-eyed people. And what strange clothing we wore!

There was also a universal fear of the hospital among the people. Operations, medicines, and treatments were unheard of. The hospital building itself was curious, since people in the region had never seen a two-story brick building. Running water was strange, electric lights were strange, and even the beds were strange. We would often find the patients sleeping on the floor, seeking a more relaxed and comfortable position. The mattresses were too soft for them. Everyday medical items, such as thermometers and stethoscopes, were new and alarming.

Obtaining permission to perform an operation was often a problem. The missionary doctor and native personnel were required to explain in simple terms and great detail the cause and need for the surgery. The staff was always friendly and reassuring. To show that we were well meaning, many times the doctor would have to allow a member of the family to go into the operating room and view the operation, as well as remain with the patient overnight. The patients were usually very grateful for everything we did for them and showed their gratitude in

---

9. This is the textbook mentioned previously in Chapter 1—see page 9; see also Appendix IV, page 185.

many ways. It was amazing the amount of pain they could stand without complaining. No narcotics were given before operations and few were given after Many minor incisions were made without local anesthetic.

I soon found that everyone was learning from everyone else. We had to learn the Korean point of view, understand their thoughts, find out what they responded to best, and then work together with faith and confidence. Because I had to organize my work without a good knowledge of the language, humorous problems could result on occasion. For example, an orderly came to me and tried to tell me something. Seeing I couldn't make it out, he took a piece of paper and drew a picture of a thermometer, then tore it in two. I got that. A broken thermometer is a common problem in any hospital. Another time I handed a nurse the medicine that the doctor had just ordered for a patient and tried to tell her, "Give this every five minutes until the patient perspires." What I actually said was, "Give this every five minutes until the patient expires." The Korean nurses, despite their usual tendency to suppress all outward signs of emotion, found this to be hilarious and laughed heartily.

Unaccustomed to the deliberate ways of the Koreans and unable to converse with them freely, I was somewhat bewildered by the formidable problem of setting up a nursing school. However, we put forth our best efforts in those early days and, eventually, things began to change. Often, just when we began to feel that our plans for training nurses were proving effective, our hopes would plunge when a promising girl decided to leave, and we would have to start over with a new girl. In spite of such disappointments, we did the best we could according to our ability and let the future take care of itself.

Each morning I would walk down the hillside from our missionary home to the hospital and look up to the great mountain that towered into the skies from the other side of the valley. Fascinated by its grandeur I would quote from Psalms: "I look unto the hills from whence cometh my strength, my help cometh from Thee, oh Lord." Later, when I had an opportunity to join a party on a climb to the top of that mountain, I felt the nearness of God, and marveling at His wonders, realized the insignificance of the petty worries of men.

As long as I was in Korea I looked forward to a time when we would be able to obtain high school graduates as trainees for nursing positions, as well as for a time when Korean girls, and all the Korean people, would learn the dignity of labor. I had great hopes, for I knew the time would come when we would have excellent nurses in Korea—nurses who would be able to stand up and take their place with the other nurses of the world. With better qualified girls, we would be able to meet the challenge and responsibility of the nursing profession. Korean girls were blessed with so many of the right personal qualities: sympathy, kindliness, and thoughtfulness. If only more American nurses were aware of the need in underdeveloped countries, and how wonderful nursing abroad is, I am sure that many more would answer the challenge and come to help with training.

Korean girls did not seem to be as athletic or as strong as our American girls. They soon become exhausted and complained of being too tired to study. I often wished I was able to furnish enough nurses to allow two to work together, because in Korea it was very common to see people working in pairs or groups. To learn more about the lifestyle and customs of the women, and to better understand my nurses, I would visit their homes with a missionary woman. At first it was difficult for me to understand why our nurses had so little endurance, but many things were made clear to me when I saw the women squatting on the floors of their little eight by eight foot rooms. If they wanted something on the opposite side, they would just roll or hunch over to it. There was no running back and forth, or up and down stairs. They did little housekeeping. They had no furniture, save perhaps a chest or two for their clothes. Their beds were mats put out on the floor at night and rolled up in the daytime. They washed their dishes with their hands and turned them upside down to dry. Observing a clock in only one of the homes I visited made it clear why our nurses had so little sense of time.

I would provide the nurses with tracts and Christian literature to show them what opportunities were available for Christian work. One day a patient converted and became a "Jesus-believing person." Two days later I heard this bedside conversation. The nurse brought a dressing tray to the patient and said, "I am going to do your dressing. 'Our Father which art in Heaven…' " The patient was repeating after her, "Our Father which art in heaven," stumbling with the words and asking to have them repeated.

There was a great need for more nurses in Korea. We hoped and prayed for the time to develop our nursing school. Visiting nurses were especially needed to follow up with cases. Patients would often leave the hospital in very bad condition, especially if they felt they were about to die. If a Korean was going to die he wanted to die at home. In the East, if you wanted to wish someone ill you would say, "I hope you die away from home." It was considered a dreadful calamity to have one's spirit wandering, never able to find its way home. In one's own home the spirit would be worshipped by family and receive sacrifices of food and clothing. We had very few deaths in the hospital as a result. Often the family gave up before we did, and would take the patient home to die. In many cases they died through lack of home care. Had nurses been able to follow up such cases, they would have been able to help comfort the patient and in some cases save a life.

Chapter 5

HOSPITAL AND OPERATION

Hospital

Koreans did not readily or willingly submit to the restrictions of a well-regulated hospital. They often wanted their family and friends with them, which cluttered the ward and interfered with our ability to provide proper care. These friends would bring quantities of hard-to-digest food and were often a nuisance, but we found that it was necessary for us to have patience with them.

"Kejung Poom" was the Korean name for a common and deadly disease among Korean children. It is essentially infantile convulsions, usually caused by intestinal irritation. Our treatment was nearly always successful, and many mothers soon brought their children to us at the first sign of the condition. At the same time, maternity cases began to increase. For a long time only boys were born in the hospital, which was a fine recommendation for the service in the eyes of the Koreans. The wife of one of our helpers finally gave birth to a girl; the spell was then broken and we no longer had that inducement to offer.

It was always difficult (and sometimes impossible) to please our patients, but that is what we strived for. We knew that a contented mind was a strong encouragement to recovery. Nonetheless, we were not without our critics. One patient left us because he said we were not clean, another because we were too clean. Some left because they were lonely, others because of a lack of privacy. Some left when we suggested operations, but others left because we refused to "cut the stomach." Most patients stayed, however, because they knew we were doing our best for them.

Hospital Life

The Korean people did not know what to do when their children and family members became ill. At times this gave the appearance of a lack of concern. For example, leaving their sick ones on the floor without even giving them a bath, combing their hair, or changing their clothes, gave an impression of neglect. One baby was brought into the hospital with pneumonia and a temperature of a hundred and three. The family thought the child was dying and had little hope for its recovery. The superstitious old grandmother had told them that if a child was taken ill before it was a hundred days old, it would surely die. The child was filthy, but we were able to show the family that with care and cleanliness, a child need not die, even if it is less than a hundred days old.

A father brought his eight-year-old blind daughter to us, and we took her in. He remained for a while, working about the hospital in exchange for her care. Since it was necessary for the child to remain in the hospital for a long period, the father eventually had to return to his home. We taught the girl the layout of the hospital, and guided by touch, she was soon able to go about freely. She did very well considering that she was in a strange building so different from her own mud and stone-walled home. In contrast, some of the older Korean women visiting the hospital were afraid to go up and down the stairs—even with eyesight! We would sometimes see them clinging to the banister and frequently they would go down sitting, one step at a time. We became very fond of the little blind girl; she became our mascot. During the few weeks she stayed with us in the hospital, the doctor performed several operations on her eyes. Her father was overjoyed when he returned and found that his daughter was able to see the gifts he had brought her and tell him their names.

On another occasion, a very sick mother arrived at the hospital, cuddling a half-starved baby. We put the mother to bed and made her comfortable. For the baby we made a formula of condensed milk and

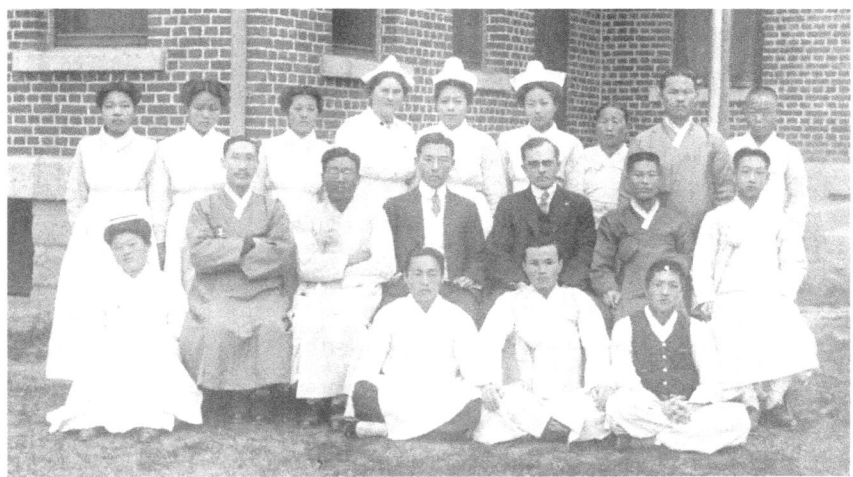

*Norton Memorial Hospital staff;
Delia is fourth from the left in the back row*

began to feed it on a regular schedule, which quickly stopped its cries of hunger. This process of artificial feeding was quite unheard of among the Koreans and attracted considerable curiosity. They were familiar with wet nurses and would feed babies rice water with a spoon from time to time, but this was a strange performance and many people stopped by the hospital to observe. They wanted to see the baby take its bottle.

Two weeks after they arrived, the mother died. The child's grandmother came by and begged me on bended knees to keep the baby until it was able to eat. Knowing that it would die otherwise, I promised to keep it for a year.

One thing would throw any Korean family into a panic: the appearance of what they called "wind disease" in their very young children. This was a condition that was usually fatal for them. The wind supposedly entered the body through the soft spot on top of the baby's head, resulting in convulsions. With the aid of prescription medication, massage in a tub of warm water, and enemas, we were able to save many of these babies. Old school Korean doctors and native grandmothers had their own special treatment for these convulsions. There was a certain weed they picked, dried, and kept on hand for emergencies. Crushing these dried leaves in their fingers, they would make a little ball, light it with a match, and when it started to burn, drop it on the soft spot of the baby's head. It did work as a counter-irritant. If the child lived, and some did, they spent the rest of their lives with a scar the size of a quarter on top of their heads. In later life this could present a problem, because Korean women always parted their hair in the middle. I noticed one who had rubbed black ink on her scalp so the scar wouldn't show.

Intestinal parasites of one sort or another plagued many of the local people. In our hospital ninety-eight percent of the patients we saw had intestinal parasites: pin worm, round worm, tape worm, hook worm, and whip worm. We routinely prescribed worm medicine for almost every patient. One disease that often undermined the health of missionaries was amoebic dysentery. We always had to be careful about our drinking water and avoid uncooked food.

The chim (needle) was used in Korea and throughout Asia as a therapeutic device. A red hot needle[10] was stuck into joints or painful areas to provide an exit for disease. Sometimes they would spit on a piece of paper, roll it up and insert it into the puncture as a drain. This treatment is known as acupuncture and has been used for millennia. It is performed with considerable ritual. The native doctors have a chart that shows many carefully chosen sites for the needles, each one for the treatment of a specific disease. Other first aid treatments were also used, such as covering wounds and painful spots with plaster, oil paper, tobacco leaves, puff-balls, snakes, and manure. Patients came to us covered with these preparations which they used to treat diseases that, realistically, could only be cured by a skilled physician.

Many Korean women suffered needlessly because they lacked the knowledge to care for themselves. Many died during confinement due to inadequate care, as did their babies. This usually occurred as a result of basic ignorance. We saw many umbilical hernias because the cord was not

---

10. Heated needles are not normally used in acupuncture. This either describes a non-standard practice or is a misinterpretation of a needle sterilization technique.

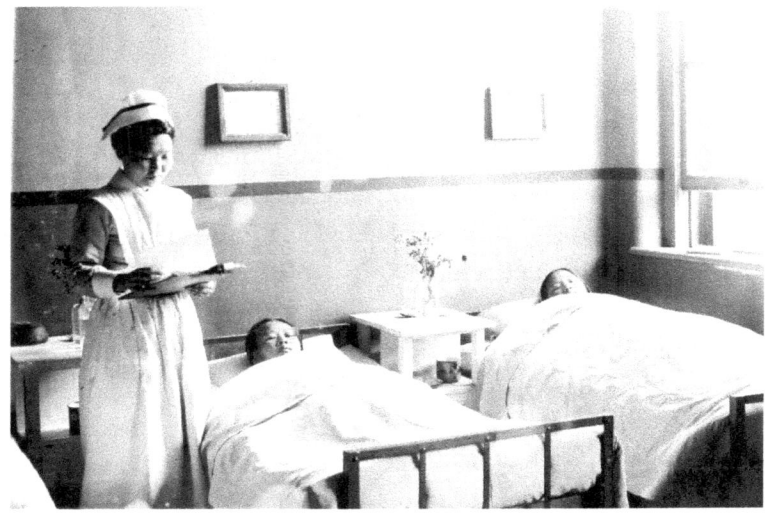

Women's ward with Korean nurse

properly cared for. A Korean superstition held that the longer the cord is left intact, the longer the baby will live. Under unsanitary conditions this resulted in unnecessary complications and infections. Women were usually up and about the day after confinement. This left them vulnerable to weariness, backache, and prolapse of the uterus. They had their own unique method for treating the latter, usually performed by the grandmother. First they would put wet cloth on the thighs. Then the prolapsed uterus would be wrapped with a cloth soaked in oil and set ablaze. When the flesh was seared, the uterus would be pushed back into the vagina. I never personally saw this done, but the procedure was described to me by a member of the hospital staff. The interior of the vagina was left a mass of scars, sometimes resulting in urinary and rectal fistulas. A ruptured uterus could then occur with conception, because the scar tissue could not expand. Many women died unless they were taken to the hospital for a cesarean section.

Korean women also suffered from a condition which the locals called Naug. Since Naug was a new term for me, I questioned one of our Korean helpers who defined it as pelvic trouble caused by a clot of blood that travels about in the abdomen. Apparently, it has one green eye. Native doctors have a remedy they use which consists of inserting a red-hot needle through the abdominal wall. If they are successful in penetrating the green eye of the Naug, the patient is cured of the disease. If they are unsuccessful, he just didn't have good luck and the patient goes on suffering. Many uterine and abdominal tumors were removed by missionary doctors using surgical techniques from patients who came to the hospital with the Korean diagnosis of Naug.

In Korea, elders occupy a position of importance and hold sway in major family decisions. From long established custom, they occupy a position of authority and respect. The oldest member of the family is the head of the household. One day a young man appeared at the hospital with a small boy, who was his brother, strapped to his back. Their mother followed several feet behind. The young man explained that his brother was very ill and that they had come because they had heard of the healing power of the missionary doctor. He had carried the boy ten miles from their small village.

We placed the boy on a bed and the doctor performed a careful physical examination. As he proceeded, he asked questions and checked symptoms. Running over his findings he recited to himself, "high temperature, rapid pulse and respiration, sharp pain in lower abdomen, tense abdominal muscles. Now we will take a blood sample and if there is an elevated leukocyte count it will mean that there is an infection." The diagnosis was clear, and the blood test verified that there was infection. "It is a pelvic abscess," the doctor stated, then went on talking quietly. "Immediate surgery is imperative, but there is no need to expect much trouble if no time is lost." After patiently explaining the procedure, he asked for permission to perform the operation. Stepping forward, the white-robed mother, who had not uttered a word previously, said "I can't agree to that." Realizing the seriousness of the situation, the doctor again tried to explain to her that surgery was the only thing that could save the child's life. Korean members of our staff also tried to convince her. In spite of the child's persistent moaning, the mother still refused. We paced the corridor and watched the crippled seconds limp by.

Finally the poor little patient, reaching a place where he could no longer endure the pain, cried out "Cut me open, cut me open." Impatient with the mother, the doctor in desperation said, "It appears that the child has better judgment than the mother." At that point the older son came to the rescue of the mother, and spoke up on her behalf; he was willing to make concessions. While it was true that women in Korea were not given much consideration, there was a time when they did receive honor: when they had a son.

"She has had four sons," said the elder brother, "and with each one has gone some of her reasoning."

Here was a woman of honor who had every right to be respected; did she not have four sons? Finally, however, something penetrated her fear and resistance, and her consent was given. There was a breathless silence as all eyes turned from the child, writhing in pain, to the doctor. A feeling of relief rippled over the anxious nerves of the medical staff and they quickly donned their surgical apparel. The operation was performed, the abscess drained, and the boy eventually walked out well and happy.

Korean assistants in the hospital were a great help to the staff as teachers and interpreters. They also assisted with the care and treatment of patients, filled prescriptions, and dispensed drugs. Most crucially, they helped the missionary doctor get his plan for treatment across to otherwise bewildered patients. The girls we were training as nurses were eager to learn and to apply their skills on behalf of Koreans who were ill, in order to help relieve their pain and suffering. We found them to be sincere, generous, courteous, and genuinely thankful to us for our efforts on their behalf. As we served with them in mutual assistance, their devotion to us grew as did our attachment to them.

The longer I remained in Korea and the more familiar I became with the people there, the more I realized that the qualities I admired in our trainees were common to all Koreans. I found them to be people of high quality and ideals, with an effective philosophy of life and a gentle, down-to-earth nature. Through our close association, I got to see and understand how they lived, how they felt, how they worked, and how they played. I came to appreciate the unique opportunity I had to get to know them.

Operation

The day a major operation was scheduled created an atmosphere of suspense among the hospital workers. On one such occasion we had a patient with a uterine tumor, so everyone was on their toes. The missionary doctor and his assistant, a Korean medical student, changed their clothes and put on their white cotton operating suits. They covered their heads with caps and their faces with gauze masks, so only their eyes could be seen peering out. The Korean nurse also wore a gauze mask and had her hair covered. Following the standard procedure, all three scrubbed their hands and forearms for ten minutes with a brush and green soap, and then plunged them into a basin of alcohol. On a table nearby was a partially opened bundle of folded sterile gowns. Slipping their hands into the sterile packets, they pulled out their operating gowns and cautiously inserted their arms. They backed up to me so I could tie their neck and belt strings and then donned their rubber gloves. In the center of the operating room, underneath our best light, we laid our patient on the table. A second Korean nurse had painted the abdomen with iodine and draped the patient with a sterile sheet with a slit in it, so that only a narrow strip of skin showed.

Acting as anesthetist, I gave the patient ether using the drip method. When I indicated that the patient was asleep, the nurse pulled a tray of sterile instruments close to the table, the doctor and assistant took their places beside the patient, and the other helpers found theirs. Once everything was ready, the doctor paused and said, "Let me pray first." As the sole physician he felt a tremendous responsibility, and prayer enabled us to enlist the support of the "Great Physician." God did bless our work and I am sure that many of those difficult operations could not have been performed successfully without His help.

Clearing his throat, the doctor extended his hand, and the Korean nurse immediately slipped his favorite scalpel into it. She was calm and alert. Seizing a handful of hemostats, she passed them to the Korean assistant. I had taught her to slap the instruments hard so that they could.

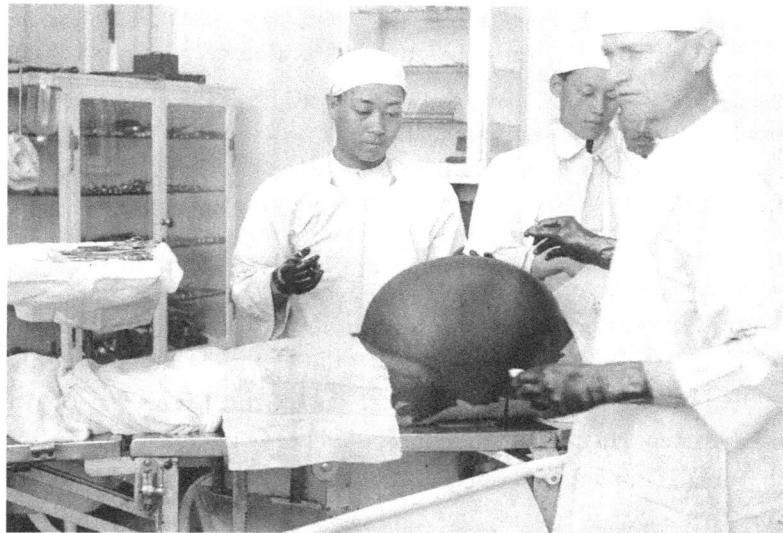

Doctor and assistants prepare for an operation

be felt through the gloved hands and she remembered my instructions There would be no fumbling or dropping of instruments during this operation. I had warned her to watch the doctor, anticipate his needs and not to wait to be asked, but to have the instruments ready. The instrument nurse is vital to a smooth operation.

As the operation proceeded, the doctor cut deftly through the skin from the umbilicus to the pubic symphysis. The Korean assistant quickly clamped the bleeders. The operation progressed layer by layer as the doctor cut, clamped, tied, and sponged. When he cut through the last layer an opening appeared, and the Korean assistant inserted his tractors. At this point the contents of the abdominal cavity could be plainly seen. Tenderly, and with utmost care, the doctor slipped his hand into the abdomen and gently brought out the uterine tumor.

We all looked and gasped. My eyes bugged out, and I stood spellbound. Here before me was one of the strangest things I had ever seen: a huge tumor. Noticing my surprise, the doctor explained that in this land, where surgery was practically unknown, tumors grew to almost unbelievable sizes. Later we found that this one weighed thirty pounds!

Clamping off the fallopian tubes, the doctor used a fresh scalpel to cut along the clamps. Then, lifting the tumor up from the cavity where it dangled with the aid of hemostats, he dropped it into the specimen basin with a clang. Tying off the clamps and suturing the stump, he checked conscientiously for bleeders. He then inspected the ovaries, appendix, and gall bladder.

"Is the sponge count correct?" he inquired.

With a nod that it was, the Korean nurse handed him a needle threaded with chromic catgut. This she did with the handle of needle holder toward him. Layer by layer, the doctor sutured his way out of the abdomen. He drew the last bit of skin neatly together with a black silk thread, straightened up and said, "This is all of my embroidery work for today."

A gauze dressing strapped with adhesive was applied to the incision and held in place with a binder. Everyone stripped off their rubber gloves and helped to lift the patient onto the stretcher. She was then wheeled back to her room and one of the nurses remained with her until she recovered. Two weeks later, with a different silhouette, the patient returned to her country home.

We saw many tumors in Korea, but not all patients were willing to have them removed. One day, a man with a large fatty tumor on his shoulder became quite indignant when the doctor asked if he would like to have it removed. "No indeed," he said "it is a blessing." Since rural Koreans at this time considered tumors to be blessings, it was easy to see why they hesitated to have them removed. They knew nothing of the many advancements which medical science had made in the battle against disease. This, coupled with superstition, kept them decidedly backward in the care of their sick.

For the missionary it meant winning the hearts and minds of the people. As Western ways began to be better understood, many operations were performed and people returned to their homes with their ailments corrected. As favorable reports spread about the foreign hospital, fear began to fade from native minds. For thousands of Koreans who had never had contact with modern medicine before, it meant a new lease on life.

Chapter 6

DISPENSARY ~ HEATHEN SUNDAY SCHOOL

Dispensary

Leaving their shoes outside, patients stepped into the dispensary waiting room, which was open every day but Sunday. In deference to Korean custom, men sat on one side and women on the other. Sitting on the floor, they waited their turn. Patients were ushered in one at a time, each with a couple of relatives or friends. It may have been curiosity or fear that brought out so many. Some had heard of the new and strange foreigners who could make people well. Some came out of curiosity, others with a sincere hope that their loved ones might be relieved of pain. It was not unusual for a man to step through the door with his wife on his back. He might have carried her as much as ten or twenty miles. Mothers and grandmothers with babies strapped to their backs could always be seen.

Various complaints brought them to the hospital. There was almost every disease and disability under the sun; the mission hospital was an excellent workplace for the general practitioner. Many cases of eye disease needed to be dealt with, including trachoma. In addition to eye problems, there were boils to open, stitches to take, fractures to set, and sprains to strap. Malaria was very common. Tuberculosis, typhoid, tetanus, and smallpox were frequently seen, and leprosy occasionally. Patients with pneumonia, Bright's disease,[11] and sleeping sickness were

---

11. An obsolete general term for kidney disease.

advised to enter the medical ward of the hospital. Those with mastoid problems, hernias, and tumors were told they would need surgery and encouraged to enter the hospital. We had to treat all of these conditions at a time when sulfone drugs and antibiotics were still unknown.

Inside the dispensary, there were work tables, shelves filled with bottles of medicine and solutions, and jars filled with gauze, cotton, bandages, and adhesive. Near one window was a unit set up for the examination and treatment of the eyes. There was also a private examining room and a pharmacy where prescriptions were filled. The fees were scaled somewhat according to the treatment and medication. No one was ever overcharged and many of the fees only amounted to five or ten cents. Our charity work was large, and a surprising number of patients paid nothing at all.

The superstitions of the Koreans were sometimes hard to overcome. For example, a mother arrived at the hospital cuddling her sick month-old baby. Through a black coating on its head we could see several abscesses. Since I was interested in the Korean approach to first aid, I inquired of our Korean helpers as to what the substance was. They told me that if a child has a rash or a spot on its body when it is born, the placenta is taken and burned. The charred mass is then mixed with oil and applied to the affected part. This treatment resulted in several bad infections, in this case to the scalp.

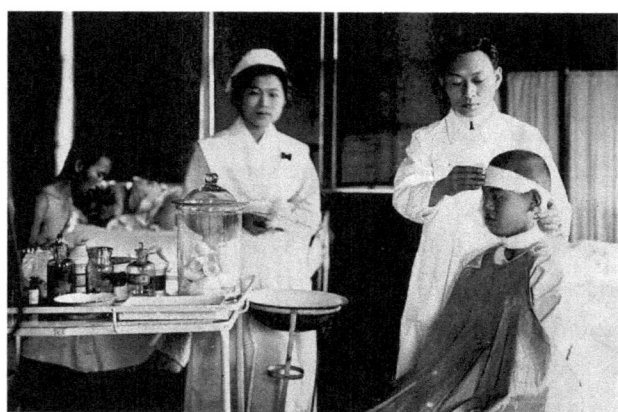

In the dispensary

After cleaning off the black mess, I took up a razor to shave off the hair in preparation for the operation. This was too much for the frightened mother.

"Don't do that," she said, "just put on some medicine and we'll go home."

The Korean assistants tried to explain that it would be far better to have incisions made in the abscesses and that the foreign doctor always wanted the skin cleaned before an operation was performed.

"Stop," she said, "I can't have anything done, for I didn't bring any money."

We assured her that we would be glad to do the operation for the baby's sake, even though she had no money. At last, after much persuading, she consented and the doctor made incisions in eight abscesses on the baby's head. When all was over, a little white capeline bandage could be seen bobbing over the blanket as the mother walked off with her baby strapped to her back.

"I just can't be operated on," another woman said, and set off for home. A half an hour later she was back. Her husband, who was undoubtedly the head of the household, had sent her back. She was able to go home for good in a couple of weeks, after having recovered nicely from her operation.

"It would be best if your wife remained in the hospital for treatment," the doctor explained to another husband. His wife objected, however, and refused to stay.

"She doesn't know anything," her husband remarked, and scooping her up on his back he carried her upstairs to the women's ward where she remained until she was well enough to go home.

One young Korean father arrived at the hospital with his sick infant. We bathed the baby, placed it in a bed, and started it on medication. To leave a sick child in a foreign hospital was apparently too much for the child's superstitious old grandmother, however. Against our advice, she came and took the child away. The father, a modern man, was indignant when he came to the hospital and found the child gone. We did all we could to prevent the child from being taken away—that domestic problem had to be solved elsewhere. Two days later, unfortunately, the baby died at home.

A man came to us one day, writhing in pain and discomfort, and was admitted. His brother was not entirely convinced that we knew the proper remedies so, just in case, he brought along a bag of dried leaves, which he meant to crush and roll into a little ball. He then intended to set them ablaze and put the little bonfires on the man's abdomen. The Koreans used this method, called moxibustion,[12] to dispel diseases. Practitioners of this method were guided by a chart of the body. Each disease had its own particular spot on the body where the fire was to be applied. We were able to hold him off and persuade him that the patient's condition could best be improved through catheterization and a good dose of Epsom salts.

A baby arrived at the hospital one day in critical condition. Unfortunately, it died while we were working to save it. The mother had brought with her a package of the medicine she had given the baby. Because she was illiterate, she had given the baby a massive overdose. At this time a Japanese company had begun flooding the country with patent medicine, some of which had reached this very rural area. I asked our Korean doctor to read the label, which was written in Japanese. It said, "The only cure for rheumatism, pneumonia, bronchitis, and cough."

To allay patient fears we would sometimes allow a member of the family to remain in the operating room. During one operation, two women appeared. Thinking it excessive to have two extra people there I asked the first why she had come. "He is my husband," she said. I gave her a place to stand where she might watch the operation, and then asked the same question of the other woman. "He is my husband too," she said. Both seemed equally concerned about him and both remained throughout the operation.

---

12. Similar to Chinese traditional medicine, Korean traditional medicine used the technique of moxibustion, or burning of processed mugwort to stimulate meridians in the body. Under conditions of normal use, moxibustion should not burn the skin but rather warm it.

One Korean family did not cease to praise us for what we were able to do for them. Their two sons had come to us with bronchial pneumonia. One was a year old and the other was five years old.

"Did you ever see children as sick as this get well?" the mother asked. I told her many had, but we must be willing to trust to the will of God. After a few minutes I returned to the room. The mother was kneeling with her head to the floor. She seemed to be praying earnestly that her babies be saved. We worked faithfully over them and both recovered, but only after a long struggle. Many turned to the missionary from desperation and said, "If you can make me well, I will examine the doctrine you teach." Medical missions were called "Christianity in action" and for many of our patients the hospital was a stepping stone to the church.

One appreciative husband brought huge bowls of Korean noodles for every member of the hospital staff, including the laundryman. He had brought his wife to the hospital because of a malformed vagina. The doctor was able to help her through plastic surgery.

One day, an elderly Korean gentleman arrived at the hospital with his son and wife and asked if we could cure his young son. The father was a typical yong-bang, a prosperous Korean gentleman who stood erect, bronzed, rugged, and proud. It is rare to find anyone who can convey a sense of dignity quite like a Korean gentleman. His balloon-like trousers were of white silk, his flowing jacket of light blue silk and he wore a black horsehair hat. The tall crown covered his grey hair, which was tied in a topknot. He walked with a strut characteristic of his class. His wife and son were also well-dressed; the ten-year old boy was a mirror image of his father, even down to his hat. His long black hair was combed up and made into a knot on top of his head—a sign that he was married.

The mother was very proud of the boy and hovered over him most of the time he was in the hospital. Beaming at him, she said to me, "He is the child of my old age." Although he was the son of the fourth concubine, the wife claimed him as her own. Sons are important for posterity in the Korean family culture. This wealthy man had spent his life hoping for a son. At last, with graying hair, his dream had come true. He was not content, however; he wanted more. He wanted to see his grandson, so he married this ten-year old boy to a much older girl.

We also had a visit from the owner of the Haeju kisaeng house. A kisaeng house is a place where female professional entertainers are paid well to sing and dance. The owner arrived at the hospital one day with a pretty young girl, beautifully dressed in brightly colored silk. He complained that he was losing money with her now because she was sickly. He bemoaned the fact that he had spent so much money on her clothes and training, so we wondered what he would do with her when he heard the doctor's diagnosis: tuberculosis!

One Korean man, who had heard rumors about the hospital, walked ten miles to the city to see it for himself. He explained to the doctor in the examining room that his food settled well on one side of his body, but not on the other. He appeared skeptical as the doctor held a little electric torch to look into his eyes, then wrapped a piece of cloth around his arm and squeezed a bulb. Next, a needle was inserted into a vein and blood was caught in a glass tube. Apprehensive, but realizing that no harm had come to him so far, he removed his shirt and watched as the doctor put rubber hoses in his ears. Following directions, he counted aloud to three as the doctor pressed a tube at various points on his chest, front and back. Odd, but a stethoscope meant nothing to him. When the examination was over, he accepted the bottle of tonic the doctor gave him, but looked inquiringly at the Korean assistant. Reassured by his countryman that the medicine was all right, and that his condition would improve if he took it, he left. Retracing his steps to his village, he soon found himself the center of attention. His cronies and all the people of the village flocked around to learn of his adventure.

"It's true," he said "the foreigners have white skin and green eyes. Some of the very young have white hair; they look old but they are not. We've always heard that foreigners steal babies and take out their eyes to make medicine, but that isn't true. Their medicine is made of salt, iron, sulfur and other things like roots, herbs, and bark." He was proud to divulge his newly found information. They marveled as he described his examination and studied his bottle of tonic with amazement.

"I take a spoonful of this three times a day," he explained.

"A spoonful!" they exclaimed. "What does it taste like? Let us try it!"

A spoon was brought and he poured out a taste all around. They smacked their lips and milled about saying, "It isn't bad at all."

Soon the patient was left standing with an upraised spoon in one hand and an empty bottle in the other.

"Oh my," he gasped, "What am I to do? It seems that if I want to get well I will have to go back to the city and get more medicine."

His demonstration and generosity were not in vain, however, for the next day the doubters and skeptics among his friends said, "We will go with you to the foreign hospital and have a look for ourselves." Unwittingly, he had helped them overcome their fear of foreigners and introduced them to Western medicine.

We offered obstetric services at the hospital, but it was slow work convincing the people to come and take advantage of them. Responding to an emergency call one night, I was led to a local home. Stepping over the door sill into the room, I encountered a sickly odor. A burning wick in a bowl of oil did little to illuminate the room. The flickering light gave a greenish look to the face of a poor woman who lay motionless on a bed. Her skin was wrinkled around pinched features and her eyes lay deep in withered sockets. Her unattended baby lay on the floor beside her. One glance told the story: hemorrhage. There was nothing that could be done to help her now. Here was another mother lost unnecessarily while giving birth.

The hospital is inevitably a place of crisis and drama, and there is a constant atmosphere of readiness and expectancy. When a distressed patient comes to the waiting room, everyone becomes very alert. Doctors and nurses step forward quickly with helping hands. The patient is carefully checked and the fight to save a life begins. If a small child has swallowed poison, its stomach is pumped. Wounds are sutured or bones set, according to need. After treatment is administered, an operation performed, or medicine given, a period of watching and waiting begins. Usually the result is relief for the patient, but sometimes it is tragic. Daily the fight goes on; the effort is unstinting. A life is precious everywhere.

Heathen Sunday School

This title may bring a smile to students of the English language; it seems such a contradiction in terms! Yet, how else to describe a Sunday school made up of dirty, noisy, wiggling half-naked boys and girls whose parents were heathens? If I gave it a less paradoxical name, you might fail to understand the colorful and dramatic scene. Here we had primitive Christian work in action.

Although missionary work had been going on in Korea for about thirty years at this time, there were many natives in rural regions of the country who had never had any contact with Christianity. Haeju, however, had a centrally located, large brick church where missionary work was well established. It had a large congregation and a well-attended Sunday school.

Since I was newly arrived, I wanted to adopt a project for my Sunday church work. I chose to teach at the Sunday school, which seemed a fitting use of my time. Since I was a medical missionary and spent most of my time in the hospital, this Sunday school served as my evangelical work. It was a benefit for me because it provided an opportunity for closer contact with the Korean people. Through it, I was able to learn a great deal more about their lives and customs than might otherwise have been possible.

The Sunday school had begun in the home of a Korean Christian. We gathered there each Sunday until attendance grew so much that we felt the need for a larger space. We searched until we found a building near the West Gate that would meet our needs. It was not a church, just a small Korean building with mud and stone walls and a thatched straw roof. There were no funds—we had not even begun taking up a collection. I offered to buy the building if the Christian men in the community agreed to do the remodeling, which they were more than happy to do.

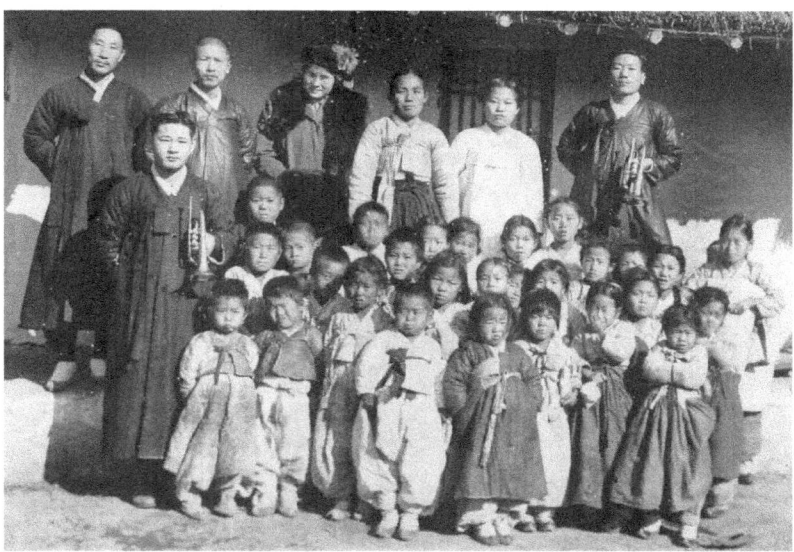

The "Heathen" Sunday School

Inner partitions were removed to make a larger room, which was constructed in a V-shape. The floor was covered with mats, and a rough pulpit was set in the corner. There was a partition down the middle of the church that separated the men from the women, and everyone sat on the floor. The Koreans, knowing how difficult it is for Westerners to sit on the floor, made me a little wooden bench. We soon had a little white-washed church for our Sunday school.

One fine young Korean man, who had been educated in mission schools, was the most active worker. One Sunday morning he took up his trumpet and played "Onward Christian Soldiers," as he walked down the street. The notes penetrated the air of the quiet town and drew a curious flock of youngsters to the street. It was a motley crowd of boys and girls, unkempt and unwashed, but dressed in bright colors. Many of the girls, and some of the boys, had small brothers or sisters strapped to their backs. The babies appeared happy in their comfortable warm seats, their little black eyes peering out of their expressionless faces. One small girl appeared to be only a couple of years older than the child she bore on her back. The little baby was contentedly eating a bit

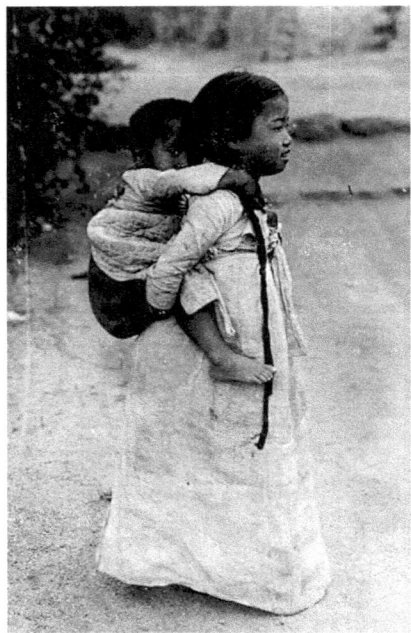

Piggy-back sibling transportation

of corn on the cob. Another baby toddled along carrying a half-eaten cucumber, closely followed by an elder sister. A few of the children staggered a bit under their human freight. The trumpeter interrupted his playing from time to time and invited them to follow and learn about Jesus. Then he struck up "Bringing in the Sheaves," and led the way to the modest, white-washed edifice where the "sheaves" were gathered in with "rejoicing."

The girls sat at one end of the room and the boys at the other. Leaving their shoes outside the door, they walked in and sat cross-legged on the floor. The young man gave the signal to rise by clapping his hands. Ignorant of the significance, newcomers were yanked to their feet with sudden rudeness by their nearest neighbor. The teacher clapped his hands again, giving the signal for silent prayer. Heads bowed and a silence of sorts fell; since this was a heathen Sunday school, one could not expect too much. Another series of hand claps signaled all to resume their seats so that the teaching of Christian songs might begin. Many of our hymns were in Korean translation. The Koreans loved them and entered into the spirit of the song, singing with all their might. Unfortunately, no one could carry a tune. No Christian in America would ever have been able to recognize the songs. We didn't care as long as they got the spirit. We would listen patiently and bear in mind the good works brought about by these small churches which were uplifting the people and spreading the Gospel. Following song time, the teacher asked a young Korean woman to teach the girls, while he taught the boys.

Is there a child anywhere who does not love a story? The faces of the audience shone with rapt attention as the teacher spoke. If a baby cried, another child would stand and teeter back and forth on its toes to quiet it, keeping an eye on the speaker with rapt attention. The children were truly learning about Christianity. On occasion the shy, giggling youngsters would laugh out loud, but most of the time they sat spellbound, captivated by the story.

Following stories there would be review questions, led by the School Superintendent. The story "The Riot at Ephesus" was told one Sunday and followed by questions such as:

"Is there any God in existence other than Jehovah?"

"No," was the answering shout.

"What are we to think of those who worship idols?"

"They are ignorant and crazy," answered an older boy.

"Who are the most deluded people in Korea?" was asked.

"Those who spit before the trees and throw a stone to the tree spirits," said a giggling young girl.

Everyone laughed at that.

"What are we to think about ancestral sacrifice and worship?" was the next question posed. This was a difficult question for children who are taught filial obedience and reverence from the cradle up.

After a brief pause, an older boy said, "That is an altogether foolish business."

"Why?" asked the teacher.

"Because our ancestors, being dead, are in God's hands, and can neither hear us nor help us." Surely heathenism was being dealt a death blow when these urchins dared to come out with such bold statements that contradicted their traditions.

These children came back Sunday after Sunday to hear the wonderful stories from the Bible. Not only were they were taught Bible stories, Christian songs, and prayers, but a few minutes were dedicated each Sunday to studying the alphabet and learning to read, since most of these children had never been to school. Many a Korean without schooling, both young and old, learned to read in the Sunday Schools.

The Koreans' everyday language is easy to learn. The New Testament and songbooks were printed in this language. Printing the Bible in the common language that all could understand, instead of their most literary style, may have contributed to the rapid spread of Christianity in Korea.

At the close of the session there were no pretty Sunday School cards to pass out to the children. However, each child received a card we had prepared by pasting a tract in the Korean language onto used postcards we had received from America.

Prizes were given to those who had brought new pupils into the school. Two little girls were shyly stepping up to receive their rewards when there was a sudden commotion on the boys' side. A boy darted out of the building, but soon came puffing back.

"Here, I've got two," he said, and marched up for his reward. This caused a burst of laughter. He was given his prize, but exhorted to bring new pupils at the beginning of class next time.

Our little church, along with hundreds of other heathen Sunday Schools throughout the country, beamed its light toward the children so that they might have the opportunity to grow up understanding the joy and peace of the Christian way of life.

Chapter 7

KOREAN RELIGIOUS LIFE ~ VISITING IN THE COUNTRY

Korean Religious Life

A Chinese gentleman was stopped by a Christian missionary who asked, "Do you believe in these gods?"

"No," was the answer, "not really, but I bow before them because a man has to have gods of some kind, and I don't know any other."

Koreans are a religious people with a sense of dependence on that which is above and superior. They firmly believe that the human and divine can find a place of intercommunication and relation, and they earnestly strive for the freedom of the soul from annoyance and pain.

The three principle religions of Korea are Confucianism, Buddhism, and Shinto. No one of these three stand out as having special or unique followers. The faiths merge into a confused jumble in the minds of most of the people; it is hard to tell where one leaves off and the other begins. A Korean might be educated by Confucius, pray to Buddha for offspring, and pay a Shinto priestess to ward off disease when ill. And so the people of Korea follow all three religions in hopes of gaining the advantages of each and thereby obtaining the greatest happiness.

Confucianism is not technically a religion, because it has no deity to worship. It is a code of ethics dealing with the conduct of human life. These are known as "The Five Principles of Conduct":

1. Blessed is the child who honors his parents, for he in turn shall be honored by his children.

2. Blessed is the man who honors his king, for he will stand a chance to be a recipient of the king's favor.

3. Blessed are the man and wife who treat each other properly, for they shall be secure against domestic scandal.

4. Blessed is the man who treats his friends well, for that is the only way to get treated well oneself.

5. Blessed is the man who honors his elders, for years are a guarantee of wisdom.

Buddhism was introduced into Korea from China three or four centuries before Christ. When Buddhists first entered, they were not welcomed by the Korean people, nor were they allowed to come within the gates of the cities. As a result, beautiful monasteries built in Chinese architectural style are found tucked away in the mountain ranges. The monks and priestesses perform daily devotions before the gods of the temple and many people from the cities travel out on foot to the mountain temples in order to worship. Buddhism makes no great distinction between the sexes. Korean history is full of incidents showing that women were equal sharers in what were supposed to be the benefits of this religion. In contrast, Confucianism is a literary cult from which women were excluded due to their lack of education. As a result, women turned to Buddhism where their devotional instincts could be nurtured. So it is said that the men are all nominally Confucians, while the women are nearly all Buddhists.

The Buddhists are courteous and hospitable and have rigid discipline; they strive to advance themselves spiritually in order to assure the best possible life in the next world. The practices that lead to this outcome are: right view, right intention, right speech, right action, right living, right effort, right mindfulness, and right concentration.[13] Their benevolence toward the old and destitute, who find peaceful asylum with them, created a certain fascination for me.

Trailing up a mountain path outside of Seoul, a group of Korean hospital staff members and I went one day to visit one of their monasteries.

---

13. This describes the "Noble Eight-Fold Path" of Buddhism.

We were served a most interesting meal of rice, vegetables, fruit, and herbs. Buddhists do not eat meat; they never kill anything. I have seen them sit and let a fly walk across their face without reaction, or tread mountain paths watching the ground at all times to avoid the possibility of stepping on an ant. Buddhists believe in the transmigration of souls.

Shinto, with its eight million gods, is a form of spirit worship. It is the most ancient of the religions and its origin is unknown. It is less a religion than a cluster of superstitions, which makes it difficult to explain. There appear to be two types of spirits in Shinto. The first is malicious, addicted to revenge and caprice. The second is kindly and brings good luck. Believers offer gifts and prayers to mollify the fiends and to persuade the kindly spirits to bestow blessings and bring good luck. They believe that the earth, air, and sea are peopled by these spirits or demons and that they inhabit the trees, shady ravines, crystal springs, and magnificent mountains. They are in the fields, by the lakes, in the bubbling rivers, and along the road. They appear from the north, south, east, and west. They are on the roof, ceiling, fireplace, and beam. They fill the chimney, the shed, the living room, and the kitchen, and are on every shelf, and in every bowl and jar. Every Korean home is populated by them; they are here, there, and everywhere. This belief in spirits keeps the people of Korea in a perpetual state of nervous apprehension, surrounding them with indefinite terrors. It is observed by all: rich and poor, high and low.

When a traveler leaves his home to set out on a journey, countless spirits waylay him. They are beside him, behind him, and whirling above him. They are crying out from the ground, in the air, and everywhere he looks. When he comes to a crude shrine, consisting of a heap of stones, he tosses on another rock to chase the evil spirits back. He then spits at the shrine to prevent the evil spirit from coming out and causing calamities for his journey. A tribute of wine, rice, shoes, or flapping string might be seen on a distorted "devil tree" on the side of the road. A newly married bride might stop on the way to her new home to tie brightly colored strips of her clothing to the tree, hoping to ward off evil spirits and encourage good ones to bring favor and sons.

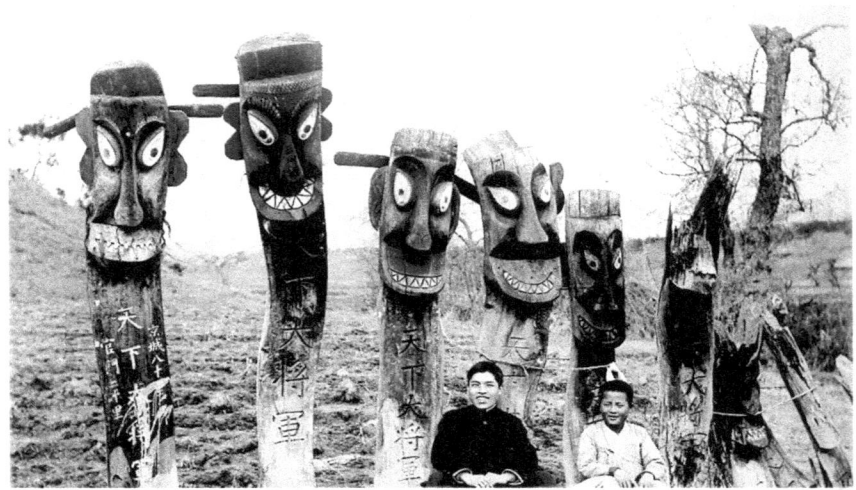

Traditional Korean janseung poles

Posts decorated with gruesome devil images[14] are seen outside many villages. On top of these high posts are crudely carved heads, the faces of which are part human and part demon. These huge grimacing faces are intended to frighten off evil spirits of disease. In the past, this was the only protection the people had during a severe smallpox epidemic.

The Korean people believe that their well-being depends on continual acts of propitiation to the evil spirits, for they are known to avenge every omission with merciless severity. The people remain bound to this yoke from birth to death and are required to make continuous sacrifices to the spirits in times of great trouble or misfortune. In their host of superstitions and fears, the Koreans know the meaning of the phrase "The devil to pay."

Sorcerers control the doings of every household. They are called in at times of birth, sickness, and death, or in the making of any important decision. They rule the land with unquestioned power. Sorcerers are

---

14. Commonly called *janseung* in Korean, these poles are similar to so-called "totem poles" in North American. They helped delineate the village boundaries and served as a focus for animist worship. Most were destroyed in mid-twentieth century modernization movements.

professionals, hired to deal with demons and appease them with offerings and gifts. The sorcerers are called upon to gain favor with the spirits and avert calamities, regardless of their fees. They supposedly possess the power of securing the good will of some spirits and averting the malignant influences of others. They do this through an assortment of magical rites, charms, and incantations. They drive out the spirits of disease to cure the sick. They predict future events and interpret dreams. They also perform exorcisms, solemn ceremonies meant to deliver a person from evil spirits or malignant influences. Their methods are quite colorful, including bright clothing and all the paraphernalia of their trade. To the beating of a drum they dance, gesticulate, and work up a real or feigned ecstasy.

Great reliance is placed on charms. Some amulets are made from the wood of trees struck by lightning, which are supposed to possess magical properties. A similar item, which I saw on occasion, was a straw doll with a coin in the body. Believing that these dolls can carry away the disease devils causing sickness in the house, these dolls are tossed out of the home and into the street.

In the district of Chairyung[15] there was a village where the people sacrificed to the spirit of a nearby mountain. They made offerings at regular intervals and every three years would sacrifice a cow. A strange thing happened one day at a home near the mountain. A calf walked off the side of the hill and onto the roof. The people who lived there managed to get it off, but a few days later it happened again. This time the people were very much concerned about the strange occurrence, so they sought a sorceress to inquire about its true meaning. They were told that it was a bad omen and meant that there would be a death in the house. This could be warded off, however, if the calf was sacrificed. These good people had always been faithful in their sacrificial services, but they didn't feel that they could afford to lose the calf. As they discussed what was to be done, they recalled a former sorceress who had become a "Jesus-believing person," and because of her new faith had

---

15. This area has not been identified in terms of its modern equivalent.

lost all fear of evil spirits. They realized that if they did likewise, they would not have to sacrifice their calf, but they didn't know how. By chance, there was a Christian hymnbook in the village that they obtained and studied faithfully. Later, when a Christian leader from a village ten li[16] away visited the village, he found to his surprise a group of people anxious to believe the "Jesus doctrine." These people listened to his instructions and accepted the word of God. From that point on, they regularly traveled the ten li to the church in the next village to worship. The missionary baptized many of these villagers into the Christian faith.

There were two new believers, a man and wife, who had a mysterious experience. One day the man saw several weasels sitting up on their hind legs near his house. This scene was very unusual so he excitedly called his friends to have a look. They talked it over in solemn whispers, shaking their heads and sucking in their breath. Such a curious occurrence must have a meaning! In the end, they came to the conclusion that this could only mean that he was to be greatly blessed and would soon become a wealthy man. Oh! How the gods had smiled upon him!

With a thrill of anticipation and picturing the moment when treasures would be his, the man felt a surge of benevolence toward the weasels. He built a little house in his yard for them and every day he would prepare rice and put it out for them to eat. Then he waited, with increasing impatience. His adventure was quite an extravagance, for he soon found that feeding weasels as well as his own family was expensive and, rather than becoming wealthy, he was becoming poor. He was filled with apprehension. What would his friends think of him now? Would they regard him as a wise man—or a fool? At last he reluctantly gave up, for he was becoming disgusted with the whole matter. Then he heard about Christianity, and both he and his wife decided to convert. After having tried out the Christian religion for a while, he invited some Korean Christians and me to visit his home.

---

16. A *li* is a traditional Chinese unit for measuring distance which was also adopted in Japan and Korea. The exact length of a *li* has varied considerably, depending on time and place. It's impossible to guess the actual distance being described here.

As we stood outside the open door, his wife gathered hats, clothing, fans, and various other things from altars they had erected to the spirits. While she was gathering these things, the man stood up and reached toward the ceiling for a strip of paper with writing on it hanging down. With a mixture of fascination and horror, he shrank from it and shuffled nervously away. The wife, with real determination, yanked it down. My interpreter read for me: "The devil is the master of this house." This paper was put with the rest of the things, gathered in a pile on the street, and set ablaze. The Korean couple gave a sigh of relief. As the items burned, one of the men prayed. Afterwards, we sang songs of rejoicing and wished the couple a long and happy Christian life. I presented them with a Korean New Testament and songbook that they brought faithfully to our little church from that time on. The wife always tried to sit next to me so I could help her find her place in these books and was ever thankful to me.

Sensitivity to a world of spirits made Koreans naturally attuned to religion. They already believed in a good spirit and an evil spirit, so when they were told who the good and evil spirits were, it was easy for them to accept Christianity. Once they became Christians it could easily be told by the spiritual radiance in their faces. There were other physical changes as well, including appearing at church washed, with hair neatly combed, and wearing spotlessly clean garments.

Ancestor worship was well-rooted in Korean culture, but it was a custom born of fear. Instead of benevolent filial piety, people lived in dread that ancestral spirits might return and do harm to their descendants. It was the province of women and children to perform the rites required to keep them at bay. On one day that has been especially set aside for the worship of ancestors, the Korean children appeared dressed in especially bright costumes. Great numbers of women carrying jars of food on their heads, with their children scampering alongside them, could be seen going up the mountainsides to where a multitude of little mounds mark the graves of the dead. I was curious to see what they would do, so one day I followed a little group up a large hill near our home. At first they did not seem pleased to have me there, but when

I told them that we did not have such customs in America and that I would like very much to see it, they allowed me to look on.

At the foot of the grave they would spread a piece of oil paper and set little dishes containing many kinds of food upon it. The children then came before the mound and bowed their heads to the ground many times as the mother took a bit of each kind of sacrificial food, broke it up, and threw it into the air for the spirits. Then the whole family gathered around and had a feast on what remained.

One young man had worn a path down several inches by walking every day to his father's grave. Mothers would point him out to their sons as an example. "See," they said, "how loyal and devoted he is to his ancestors."

It is essential in ancestral worship to have posterity. Every man arranges to have his son married as early as possible, so that he might see his grandson before he dies. If a man fails to have a son by his lawful wife, he takes a concubine. Every man seeks to assure himself while he is still alive that there will be someone in the family line to carry on the sacred rites of ancestor worship.

Occasionally, I was able to go with a native Christian woman to visit in the homes of the community. I would wear low shoes without ties for this house-to-house visiting so I could step out of them easily before entering the house. Many times I looked out and could see youngsters trying on my shoes.

"Is the mistress at home?" the Christian woman would call out. The paper door would slide open and we would be invited in. In many homes we found altars erected for the worship of ancestors upon which could be found beautifully made clothing, shoes, and bowls of food. A tablet with the names of the family members is hung on the wall, and great respect and honor is shown to this tablet for it is supposed to contain the spirits of the departed. On certain anniversary days, food is set out for the spirits before the tablet and ceremonies are performed.

Some non-Christians received us willingly and listened with interest, while others paid no attention to us. In the homes where we had been invited in, we sang hymns and the Christian woman would explain something from the Bible and lead a prayer. We would invite the lady to attend church and send her children to Sunday School. In spite of the medley of superstitions and variety of religions present, Christianity has made progress more rapidly in Korea than in any other Asian country.

Visiting in the Country

Wishing to know something of the rural life and also to see something of the work of other missionaries, I decided to take a trip into the country. The evangelical missionary with whom I shared a home often spent several weeks at a time visiting the rural people. On one such occasion, when she was planning a short, three day-trip to several of the interior villages, I decided to accompany her.

Her cook arranged for a jiggy man to carry our supplies and bedding. In this country most moderate-sized loads are carried on the backs of men. Bullock carts are used in cities, but country roads are little more than paths worn deep by the feet of generations of men and women walking over the country laden with heavy burdens. The roads were slightly convex and the rain drained off into the curbed ditch, which also served as an open sewer.

We traveled several miles in rickshaws until we had to turn off the main road. From there we proceeded on foot toward the village, walking on narrow paths between muddy rice paddies. We learned that all freight and produce had to be brought in and out of the villages on the backs of bulls or pack ponies on these narrow paths.

Farms we passed contained no single homes; the people who work them all lived in houses clumped together in little villages. We were told that the homes were built huddled together to provide protection from wild animals. We were also told that the land was owned by absentee landowners and that each farmer lived in the village, going out daily to work on his allotted portion of land. These were typical Korean homes, only a little more crude. In the cities there were many roofs of heavy black tile, but here the roofs were thatched rice straw, held down with ropes. Walls were the usual stone and mud, and houses were shaped like a horseshoe, with a door at the end opening into the road. There was a court in the middle, which was usually covered with flagstone. Sometimes there would be a small flower patch in the middle.

The country people also dressed in the native white garb, but were not quite as clean as their city cousins. Their white garments were dark with dust. Their faces wore expressions of concern and their skin was dark and leathery from long exposure to the sun.

In some of these villages there were small churches where the people could gather on Sunday to study the Gospel and learn the principles of Christian living. A circuit preacher with training from the City Bible School or Theological Seminary would often have five or six of these little village churches to care for. He would also have a clan leader or strong Christian worker in each church, then he himself would visit and preach. These churches and preachers were under the jurisdiction of the general missionary board. The lady missionaries visited the churches to work with the women. Here in the mission field we found that the religious teachers spent time living among the people, learning to know them intimately and sharing something of their daily lives.

The villagers had received word that missionaries were coming that very day. As we walked along we encountered a group of women who had come out a long distance to meet us. They gave us a hearty welcome and walked back with us into the village. They had known for some time that we were coming, yet had prepared no room for us. As we stood and talked, I could see clouds of dust being swept from a room. As I watched it swirl out, I had a twinge of apprehension about what I would find and rather shrank from going inside. When they took us to our room, the door slid open and we stepped up over the sill. The room was absolutely bare, with no furniture or pictures. It was a typical Korean room, eight feet square with a low ceiling. The walls were papered white and the stone and cement floor was covered with the usual Korean oil paper. The cook put up our cots, made our beds, and opened our folding chairs. We had our own candle for the night. Many Korean homes had only a rolled wick in a small cup of oil for light.

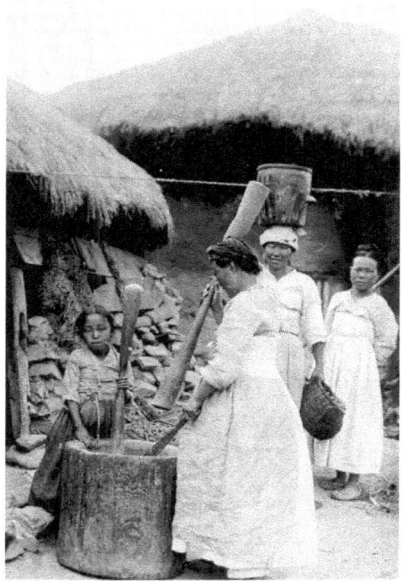
In the countryside: Korean women and girl

In the evening we carried a lantern to the church, since there were no other lights in the village.

The cook knew how to prepare American food and made our meals for us from supplies he brought, which included water from a spring for tea and for washing. He cooked on a charcoal brazier in the courtyard, bringing the food and tea to us on a tray. As we ate and got settled in, we noticed that we were surrounded by a crowd of curious Koreans, standing and watching. They were motionless; black eyes shifting occasionally in expressionless faces. With some impatience, we slid the door shut. Plenty of light came through the translucent latticed paper door and windows.

"Privacy at last," I thought. But when I chanced to glance toward the window I froze at what I saw. There was a hole in the paper and a black eye was peering through. What the people did was wet their fingers, put them against the paper and bore holes to peek through. As I watched there was another and another. How creepy, uncanny, and weird it was to have all those eyes peeping at us!

My companion quickly rose to the occasion. She was used to traveling in the country and had come prepared. From out of her supplies she drew forth a piece of thin red cloth which she hung over the broken door and windows so the eyes could no longer see inside. Later, when I asked about the toilet, I was told I would have to go to the cow stable. I never dared to think of how many eyes might have followed me there!

The villagers were friendly and kind throughout our stay. My friend had staunch supporters among the native Christians. Her many visits to the village had helped her to gain their general confidence and good-will. Her work included an afternoon meeting with the women at the church, which consisted of prayer, Bible study, and instructions on Christian living and conduct. Many of our Christian hymns have been translated into Korean; the women loved them and would sing them with fervor, even when they were unsure of the tune.

After the meeting she had interviews with the women to discuss their personal problems. Then she would take some time to visit in non-Christian homes, accompanied by a native woman who was well-versed in the Bible. Later, in the evening, she held another worship service for all the women of the village who were interested. Christians who regularly attended church brought neighbors and friends.

At the afternoon meeting it was announced that I was a nurse and would be willing to see anyone in the village needing medical attention. I set up my clinic in the courtyard and proceeded to treat those who came. I was well supplied for the task because I had brought along dressings, alcohol, iodine, ointment, aspirin, and cathartics. Two cases were more severe than the others. One man had a face that was swollen and red. Studying it for a few minutes, I noted a strong line of demarcation. "Erysipelas,"[17] I thought. I explained that I did not have the medicine with me to treat that condition, but that he could get help in the city at the Missionary Hospital. He heeded my advice and eventually got relief for his condition from the missionary doctor there. Another man had experienced severe pain in his abdomen for more than twenty-four

---

17. Erysipelas is a type of skin infection caused by streptococcus bacteria.

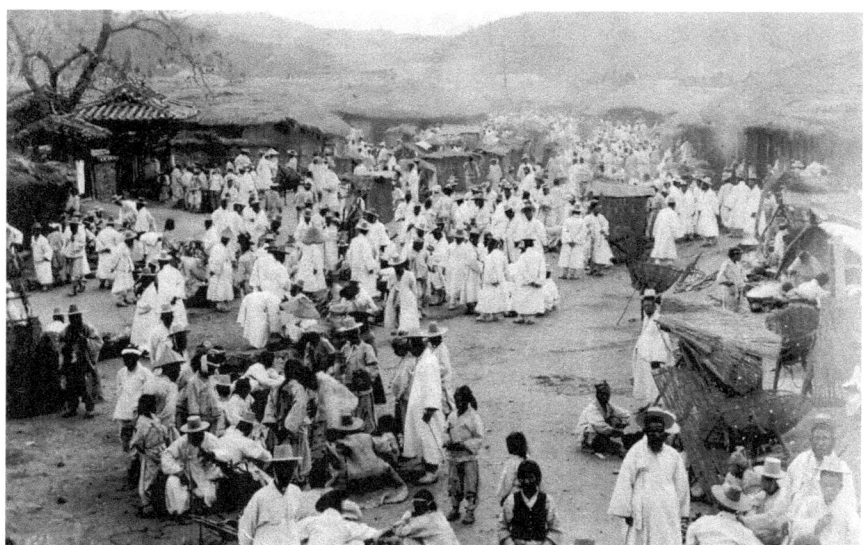

Korean village market

hours. His symptoms suggested a need for surgery, and I recommended that he go to the hospital as well.

I then visited several very ill patients in their homes. One man, with considerable edema,[18] appeared to have a nephritic and cardiac condition. I couldn't help him with first aid. His case appeared to be hopeless, and I doubted whether any doctor would be able to help. I was sorry he had not come to us months before.

We continued to be a curiosity in the village. Sometimes women would reach out and just touch me. Some took my hand and examined my skin, because it was so different from their own. Old grandmothers were the boldest; they would touch my breasts and say, "You surely must feed your babies very well." I couldn't explain that I wasn't even married. Who ever heard of a grown woman not being married?

On the third morning we started for home. This time we took a different route so we could visit other villages on the way. In the first, we

---

18. An abnormal accumulation of fluid beneath the skin or in body cavities; the author here associates this symptom with advanced kidney and heart problems.

happened to arrive on their weekly market day. There are no shops in these small villages and so the only opportunity the people have to buy anything is on market day, which brightens their otherwise dull lives with activity and color. Peasants bring whatever they have to sell or barter: some fowls in coops, pigs, homemade straw shoes, wooden spoons they had whittled, and rice. Market day is a day of excitement—there is the thrill of bargaining and the opportunity to spend the day with neighbors and friends.

In these villages there are no movies, radios, or television. There are no books or newspapers, no cars to drive, and nowhere to go. Participation in market day is therefore an important element in the social life of the community. The villagers gossip and the peddlers bring news from the outside world. Peddlers are well-dressed and respected merchants who travel regular circuits on set days. They either carry their goods on their backs or employ jiggy men to carry them. They display their wares on mats spread out on the ground. Such everyday items as pipes, tobacco pouches, combs, dyes, silk cloth, silver hair pins, oil paper, writing paper and brushes, food bowls, iron cooking pots, peanuts, chestnuts, persimmons, dried fish, and many other essentials of Korean life can be found. Each peddler squatted beside his mat. As a buyer came up I listened to them as they bartered back and forth, beating each other down. I observed that to both the buyer and the merchant bargaining was a fine art. For me, it was an interesting scene to observe, but I had no desire to participate.

We visited three more small villages on our return journey, stopping briefly at each. They were all much alike, with one to three hundred curious people in a village. Occasionally a mangy, half-fed, mongrel dog would step forward looking for friendliness. One village we had to bypass. It was a sad thing, because they had once had a strong Christian leader there to carry on the work. When he became a backslider, it left the village leaderless and now there was no missionary work conducted there.

Once my companion had finished her business, we would start on our way again, following the paths between the rice fields. As we walked, we

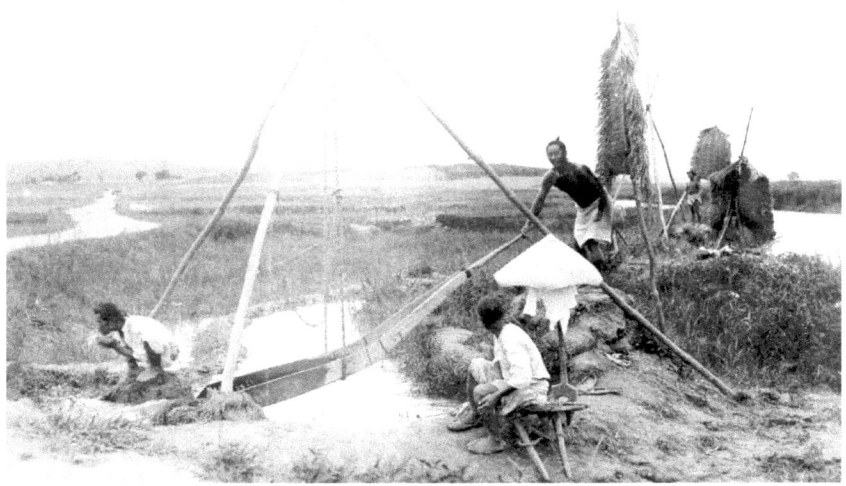

Korean irrigation system

noticed that the simple method of irrigation that Korean farmers used in their rice fields was very effective. It allowed the fertile valleys to be intensively farmed. The ground was cultivated by crude plows pulled by oxen, and in these irregular, muddy paddies, families rolled up the legs of their cotton trousers and planted their rice seedlings.

When we reached the main road, the cook was able to hire a couple of ponies for us to ride back to Haeju. In three days we had traveled over a hundred miles, mostly on foot, and visited five villages. Very much in need of a bath, we were glad to get back home.

I was grateful to have had this experience with Korean farm people. I could see what a sturdy, stalwart, and hard-working people they were. But most of all I returned with great admiration for the missionaries, who spent day after day for months at a time, carrying the message of Christ into the deepest parts of the country, showing the way to salvation for unbelievers, and inspiring and teaching those who had already become Christians. Did the faith of these converts falter and die out? Was it just a fad to follow the Westerners and accept their religion? After being converted, did they adhere to Christian practices or slip back into superstition? Koreans had always believed in good and evil spirits. When they were told that there is one true God, a God of love, they understood and accepted it. They well knew that there were evil spirits abroad in the world, so it was a relief to discover that they no longer needed to make sacrifices to buy them off. Some who accepted Christianity undoubtedly slipped back. Some were "rice Christians" who professed belief for the material gain they might receive from contact with Westerners. But most were genuine converts with deep religious experiences, who became great students of the Bible and attended church regularly. Their sincerity can be understood by the fact that Christianity has spread more rapidly in Korea than in any other country where missionaries have gone. There are many small churches throughout rural regions, and in Seoul there is a Theological School for training Christian leaders. Koreans are steadily developing their own Christian leadership and identity.

Chapter 8

KOREAN SCHOOL ~ NATIVE WEDDING ~ NEW YEAR

Korean School

As I walked along a narrow rocky street in Haeju, noise from a building attracted my attention. It was an old-time schoolroom located in the teacher's home. The boys had left their shoes outside and were seated on the floor on highly polished oil paper. They sat cross-legged and swayed back and forth, shouting out their lessons, repeating them over and over as a means of memorization. This made the school very noisy—the din could be heard many blocks away. If a boy stopped shouting, the master would tap him on the shoulder with a stick. Through persistence and diligence, they were able to memorize classics of Korean literature.

Until mission schools were founded, girls and the poor received no formal education. Boys from wealthy families, however, were taught to read and write in the Chinese language. The Chinese, Korean, and Japanese languages all use the same characters for writing, but pronounce them differently. Since the foundation of the Korean language is Chinese, educated Koreans know thousands of Chinese characters. When they write, they paint the characters with a brush and black ink. For a long time only scholars could read and write. In the fifteenth century, a phonetic alphabet was created with simplified characters. It had eleven vowels and ten consonants. Called Hangul, it was written vertically from right to left in the Chinese manner.

By the time I arrived in Korea there were already many government schools, although education was not compulsory. Christian missionaries had made day schools available for girls and boys throughout the country. In large cities high schools had been established, and some students had the opportunity to go to school from kindergarten through college.

Native Wedding

Returning from church one Sunday, I stopped to watch a marriage ceremony being conducted in the street in front of a house. A large number of people had gathered under an awning and were seated on mats on the ground. A table in the center held paper flowers, candles, fruit, nuts, and wine.

The bridegroom, a boy of sixteen, was dressed in native ceremonial wedding garb, and stood at one end of the table. His hair, which usually would hang in a long black braid down his back, was collected in a "topknot," over which he wore a black horsehair hat. Marriage confers respect, and from now on his voice would be acknowledged among men, despite his youth. He would now be addressed with full honorifics, for on his wedding day he becomes a man. He held a piece of cloth before his face that allowed only his eyes to be seen.

The bride, a girl of fourteen dressed in gay colors, was led out of the house by two women. Her hair was well-oiled and decorated with many brightly-colored flowers. The hair on her forehead had been carefully plucked out, leaving a high, square forehead. Her face was covered with whiting, her lips were painted red, and a bright red spot was painted in the middle of her forehead. Her hands were covered with long silk bags, tied around the wrist, which she held up over her face during the ceremony.

The bride and the groom bowed to the ground before each other several times. Then a cup of wine was passed between them six times. After the passing of the wine, they bowed again—the bride three times and the bridegroom twice. The bride was then led back into the house, where she would be honored, for this was her day of days. A great feast was to follow, and back in the house I could see many tables of food. The men would sit down together, while the women remained by

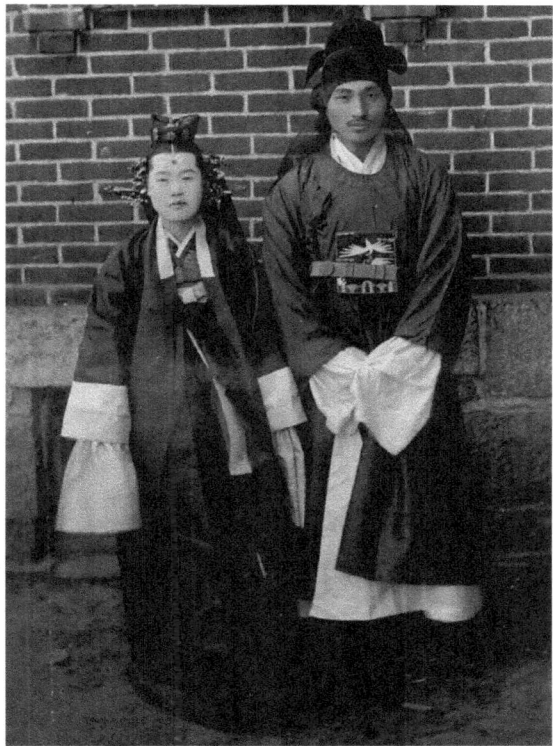

Korean bride and groom

themselves. When the wedding ended, the bride would be carried to her new home in a closed chair on the shoulders of four men. She would go from the seclusion of her old home to the seclusion of her new one. In the upper and middle classes of Korean society, this seclusion is nearly total. Upper class women never go out by daylight except in completely closed chairs. They may go out with a lantern at night and visit with friends, if attended. With the coming of Western influences, this strict seclusion shows signs of slowly giving way, even among the upper classes.

Later, my Korean friends explained the marriage customs of the country to me. I found it remarkable that young couples do not choose each other. I was surprised to learn that marriages are arranged by the father of the groom, whose duty it is to provide a wife for his son. He seeks the best prospect possible, often employing a go-between. A prospective bride's disposition and health are considered, and a sample of her sewing is inspected. In Korean homes all the clothes for the family are made by the women, so daughters are expected to learn to sew. They learn the skill from their mother and in order to please her, they produce beautiful needlework. They must, because one day a sample will be sent to a prospective bridegroom's home.

The bride and the bridegroom have little to say about the whole matter and frequently have never seen each other before the day of the wedding. They consent as a matter of course. A Korean girl would be lost if she were told to find a mate on her own. Marriage is a family affair, and parents give a great deal of consideration to the task of choosing the best match. On the whole, these arrangements work well. The practical side of married life is accounted for, and passion can develop over time. Wives stay busy with babies, food preparation, washing, and ironing, all of which consume a great deal of time. Wash day, for example, starts with ripping up all the seams of the garments. The pieces are boiled in lye and carried to a nearby stream where they are swished and rinsed in the water, then beaten on a stone with a wooden ladle. After this they are spread out in the bright sun to bleach. The clothes will then be dampened, folded, and then ironed by beating on a flat stone with two sticks. The pieces are beaten to a beautiful luster. The rat-a-tat sound of Korean ironing sticks is highly characteristic. It can be frequently heard late into the night. After ironing, all garments are stitched back together.

Marriage usually takes place at the age of seventeen or eighteen, although I have seen married boys as young as ten or twelve. In most of these youthful marriages the girl is older, in hopes of there being sons as soon as possible. The accepted custom is that the oldest son takes care of his parents for the rest of their lives when they get old. As a result, every father wants to see his grandsons before he dies, to ensure that his old age is not a time of insecurity, but one of peace and happiness.

The groom's father sends the material for the bride's wedding dress. There is no dowry or exchange of money, but the bride takes with her a large trousseau of beautifully made clothing that will last a long time.

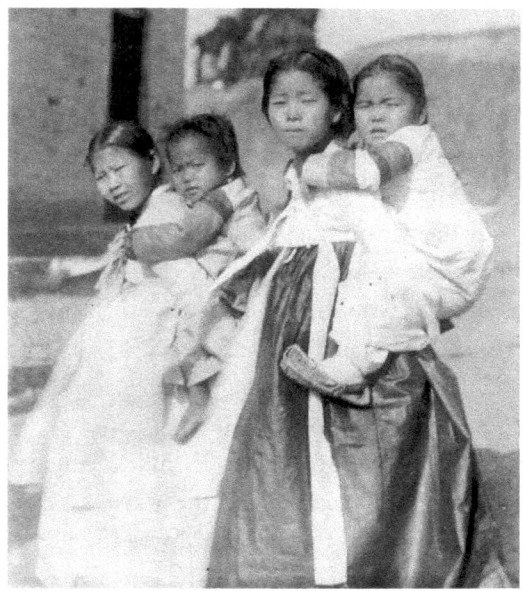

Korean girls with younger siblings

It is packed in a handsome marriage chest of polished wood with brass clamps and decorations.

What does this wedding day mean to the bride? Up to the age of seven girls play with the other children of the household and neighborhood. At the age of seven, however, they are taken into the seclusion of the women's quarters, which is one privilege that women have: complete privacy in their part of the house. It is considered sacred. No trespassing is allowed. When they move into the women's quarters of their new homes, young brides are dominated by their mothers-in-law, who expect their daughters-in-law to help with the work and to bring more sons into the family. In whatever she does, however, a wife must have the consent of her husband, for she is his slave. She must accept his edicts in silence and attend to his every need. He can beat her or treat her with respect, but he would be mocked and lose respect if he showed her any outward affection or treated her as a companion.

I have watched very young girls at play. Often, they will make a little roll of cloth and put it on their heads. On top of that they place a small stone and walk about, trying not to let it fall. In this way they practice balancing and learn the art of carrying things on their heads.

When they become teens, these girls appear happy, despite never having the types of experiences that Westerners associate with that age group. Dates with boys, dancing parties, and picnics are unknown. Etiquette forbids them from associating with boys and men. They do not grow up in idleness, however. From earliest childhood they are trained in the duties of wife and mother. It is not considered necessary to teach a girl to read or write but she is taught to wash, cook, and sew. They spend their time cooking, washing, ironing, sewing, embroidering, and caring for and playing with the babies.

Gossip in their world is indulged to its fullest extent; there is little they do not know of what's going on in the household, neighborhood, or village. When I visited in their homes I was usually entertained by the mothers-in-law, but I could see pretty young girls peeking through cracks or partially open doors. They don't miss a thing. Not one can read or write, but they are hardly ignorant, though they may lack such information that men glean from reading newspapers about wars and earthquakes. They know all about theft, adultery, betrayal, when the next baby is due, and which husband has summoned a wife to his room.

Early lessons for young girls include the three obediences: as an unmarried girl to her father, as a wife to her husband, and as a widow to her son. She meekly and demurely accepts the superiority of men. In Korea, the man is the ruler of the family. His word is law and his decisions must be accepted. A wife must show her husband respect. Their relationship must be harmonious; the husband active, the wife passive. They are never demonstrative. One never sees them kiss each other. Although a Korean father loves his children very much, he does not show a great deal of affection. Rather, his attitude is very dignified, and the children must show him the proper respect. Children are very polite when they speak to their father. Rarely does one see a child who is out of control.

When a Korean woman becomes the mother of a son, her position is greatly improved; she receives enhanced stature and respect. The more sons she has, the more respect she receives. The family system provides a form of security. Nobody gets ahead but nobody starves so long as there are living relatives. Distant relatives may appear suddenly and join the household. They cannot be turned away for it is the understood duty of the head of a family to provide assistance. This creates a drain on resources which slows the system and has its disadvantages, but for the security of the dependent, it is a blessing.

Americans are shocked by arranged marriages and polygamy, as well as the understanding that a widow and her children are inherited by the deceased husband's male relative. In the Korean social system, however, there are usually no unprotected widows, orphans, or old maids. Women may lack freedom of choice and have a hard time in some ways, but they are not left to fend for themselves. If they lose their husband through misfortune, they are not cast adrift.

One day a sick woman arrived at the hospital in a flurry of commotion. "She is at the point of death," the family said. Appraising the situation a little more calmly, we took her to the delivery room and soon announced the birth of a daughter. The woman's mother-in-law dropped to the floor upon hearing the news. Not in a faint as I first thought, but in perfect disgust. She soon rose to her feet, and although the process of labor was still incomplete, she started to abuse the poor young mother. She rattled on about how much the household had done for her, how much work they had saved her, and how well they had fed her. "Now, what is our reward?" she asked. "You've given us nothing in return but a girl."

In this land where sons are so precious, it seems that there is very little welcome for girls. I turned to my Korean nurses and said, "What's wrong with girls? Are we not girls?" They looked at me in mute silence and seemed to be thinking "What a strange person you are, not to accept the superior value of a son." The importance of sons in the family can only be understood in the context of Korean reverence for ancestors, because only sons can continue the family line.

This poor little newborn girl might not even receive a name. She might be called little pig. For years she may be known as Wong's daughter.

When she is married she will be known as Paik's wife. Then when she bears a son she will be called Kim's mother for the rest of her life. Perhaps hinting at a sign of changing times, however, some pretty names are now appearing, such as Pear-Blossom-as-She-Grows.

The rhythmic crying of paid mourners would indicate a house where a death had occurred. There were no burials within the city gates; all grave sites were on the sunny slopes of open hillsides. One day I watched a woman who had been hired by a family to choose a fitting spot for a grave. Followed by members of the family, who anxiously awaited her decision, she ran ahead, turned to the right, hesitated, retraced her steps, and turned left. She looked like a sorceress conducting an exorcism. After keeping the family in suspense for some time, she pointed out a spot she considered an appropriate resting place that would give peace to the departed and comfort to the family. They gratefully paid her fee and buried their dead relative with much dignity. Many bodies were wrapped only in cloth and buried without a coffin. Stone figures and tablets were sometimes erected to mark the grave.

Mourning often extended for a long period of time. Mourners could be recognized by their clothing. We frequently met them on the street dressed in sackcloth and wearing a robe made of straw-colored hemp cloth. On their head they wear a woven straw hat that looked like an umbrella and was sometimes as much as four feet in diameter. They would use a screen, made from about six inches of sackcloth, which they would hold in front of their face as they walked along.

New Year

Korea uses a moon-based calendar; the New Year begins in February. Korean New Year is a most interesting holiday. Everyone cleans up and dresses nicely, especially the children, who look like little rainbows dressed in clothes made of a variety of the brightest colors. Men and women dress mostly in white, though some also appear in colors. Pale blue is a favorite color among the women and men often wear blue or purple pants.

Everybody has a bath, for New Year is the annual bath day; it is also the annual birthday as well as the annual pay day. Koreans record their age according to the number of New Years they have observed. For example, a child born in January would be a year old on New Year's Day, although we would only consider him a month old, and the next year would be called two because he has passed two New Years, although in our system he is only a year old.

On each New Year, Koreans try to pay off all their debts, and if they can't, new promissory notes must be made out. It is also a time of feasting and much food is prepared. Early in the morning on New Year's Day they worship their ancestors. Later in the day, younger men go calling on their elders and neighbors to give each the New Year's greeting, which consists of bowing to the ground. In any given group, the oldest member is greeted first because age is venerated.

The New Year's holiday is observed for an entire week. On certain days during this period women are not seen at all on the street, although other days are set aside for them to visit with friends and relations. Korean girls have a special game for this time of year which they call "teeter-totter." A board is placed upon a block about a foot high. They do not sit on the board like American children do with a seesaw, but stand up on it and jump. When a girl on one end comes down, the girl on the other end of the board springs three or four feet into the air. It appears to be a great sport.

The Korean New Year seems to include all of our holidays in one. It has feasting like Thanksgiving, gift-giving like Christmas, and bright new clothes like Easter. It also resembles birthday parties, since it represents every Korean's birthday.

Chapter 9

LIFE IN KOREA ~ THE FIRST WORLD WAR ~ CHANGCHUN ~ HARBIN ~ REFUGEES

Life in Korea

Korea is a land of beautiful mountains, waterfalls, rivers, and valleys. In springtime, dark green evergreens make a splendid contrast to pink azaleas. The summer is lovely too, when forsythias fade and bright summer flowers bloom. But summer brings with it humid, almost tropical heat, which we found debilitating. The sun's rays were most trying and we found it necessary to protect ourselves from it by wearing dark glasses and pith helmets, carrying sun shades, and avoiding going out in the heat of the day altogether. Often, when we did go out, we would put a wet handkerchief underneath our hats. Those who failed to take precautions against the sun ran the risk of severe headaches or even sunstroke.

In addition to the terrible heat, summer was also the rainy season, which made it an exhausting time. A curtain of clouds often hid the mountains, which made everything grey and dark. One even felt the sound of water. One summer it rained and rained for days and days, almost continuously for a month. Everything was reduced to a hopeless state. Books, shoes, and gloves molded, and our clothes rusted on their hangers. Doors became so swollen with moisture that we could not even close them. Our dresser drawers stood open. Our salt stood in little pools in the salt dishes. Envelopes stuck together and stationary was ruined. Bedding became damp and the floors were covered with mold. The heat and humidity sapped the vitality from the hardiest souls.

Everyone showed signs of languor and exhaustion. Robbed of energy, our spirits became dampened too. Just when we got to the point where we could stand it no longer, the sun came out bright and strong. Rugs, bedding, and clothing were hung on clotheslines, books were dusted and shoes blackened. Once more we took a new lease on life.

In those early days there were few options available to beat the heat. Electric fans, refrigerators, and air conditioners were as yet unknown in Korea. Early missionaries would escape the city for vacations on the coast. There were two fine summer resorts: Wonsan Beach[19] on Korea's east coast by the Sea of Japan, and Sorai[20] on the west coast by the Yellow Sea. Many of the older missionaries owned their own summer cottages and others were available to rent.

The summer season, while a time of rest, did not mean inactivity. There was tennis and swimming, and for rainy days, games and stunts. Planning sessions for the year's work also took time. There were meetings which gave the missionaries an opportunity to compare notes with their fellow workers, to talk about common problems, and to work out policies and plans.

It was a period of physical and spiritual refreshment for many missionaries, especially those who had spent much of the year in lonely rural stations, completely out of touch with the outside world. It was an opportunity for various people to get together, such as members of different mission groups and business and professional people. On Sunday there would always be a non-sectarian church service, each conducted by a missionary from a different denomination.

Under the incredibly blue skies of autumn, Korea would reveal some of her artistic beauty. The gourd growing up the side of the house showed its green leaves spread out over the rounded thatch roof, and

---

19. Wonsan is still a popular beach resort for North Koreans.

20. The name "Sorai" seems to no longer be in use. It is mentioned in the writings of many American and European missionaries serving in Asia in the early twentieth century. Sorai is described as a "village" in northern Korea, in the Yellow Sea Province, and was considered the "cradle of Korean Protestantism," having been evangelized by a native Christian convert as early as 1884.

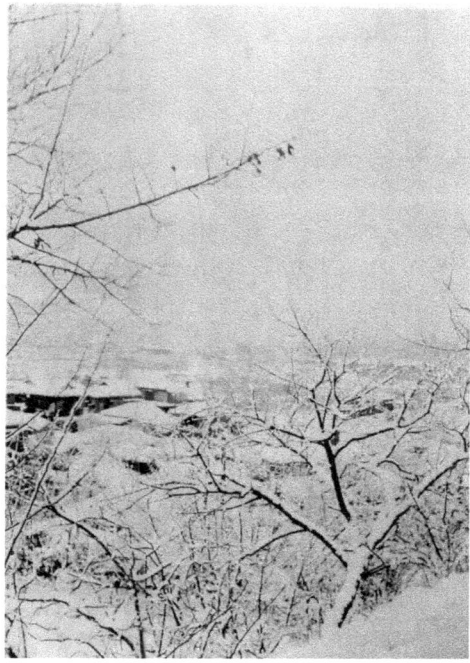

Korea in winter

yellow gourds hung from their vines. On a portion of the roof, bright red peppers were placed in the sun to dry.

Winter brought exhilaration, and people quickened their step. The air was sharp and thin, dry and chilled. The wind, clear and knife-edged, would often bring snow. Mountaintops were first to be blanketed, then the snow would fall steadily and soundlessly through the valleys until the little mushroom-shaped houses looked like a flock of sheep huddled together. The rivers froze completely and gave an opportunity to skate for those who knew how.

Koreans dressed for the cold in clothes made with a padding of cotton between two layers of material. Some wore hats or ear muffs and tucked their hands in the opposite sleeve to keep them warm. The snow storms would not last long, and the winter soon passed. Then the hopeful New Year would arrive, when the whole world would break forth again in all its natural beauty.

The First World War

The First World War was more than an historical event. It was a deeply personal and emotional experience for all who lived through it—overseas or at home. Though the war was acute in Europe, its drumbeats were far away for us at first. The ominous undertone, the rumble of war drums, was heard in America only as distant echoes. It was just another European brawl from far across our protective ocean. Americans felt safe and secure. We talked about the war and looked on with pity and horror, but the struggle was not ours. We were observers only. But then, inexorably, the roll of the drums became louder and closer until suddenly we found our safety and isolation were gone.

Korea was quiet and little disturbed by the Great War. For Americans living there, however, there was an alertness that moved into action. One local Red Cross Society sponsored a Liberty Loan drive and great quantities of dressings were folded by the ladies. When the United States entered the war, it presented a challenge for young missionaries, who asked themselves: "Should we remain in Korea, or should we return home and take part in the war?" The nurses in my hospital had a Red Cross unit in Europe. I had a persistent feeling that I should return and join the Presbyterian Hospital Unit, but our Bishop helped change my mind. Speaking before a group of missionaries, he assured us that we could not serve our country in any better way than to continue with what we were already doing—our daily mission work. This, he said, showed the good will of the United States toward the country we served and a person-to-person friendship between the citizens of our country and theirs. It was a "hands across the sea" type of thing. Reassured that our missionary work was also patriotic work, I was content to remain. Nonetheless, I made up my mind to be ready for any emergency or local disaster, little dreaming the call would come so soon.

During the heat of the summer I took a month's vacation at the sea shore with other missionaries. The year before I had gone to Wonsan Beach; this year I vacationed at Sorai Beach. I was there, in August, 1918, when the call came.

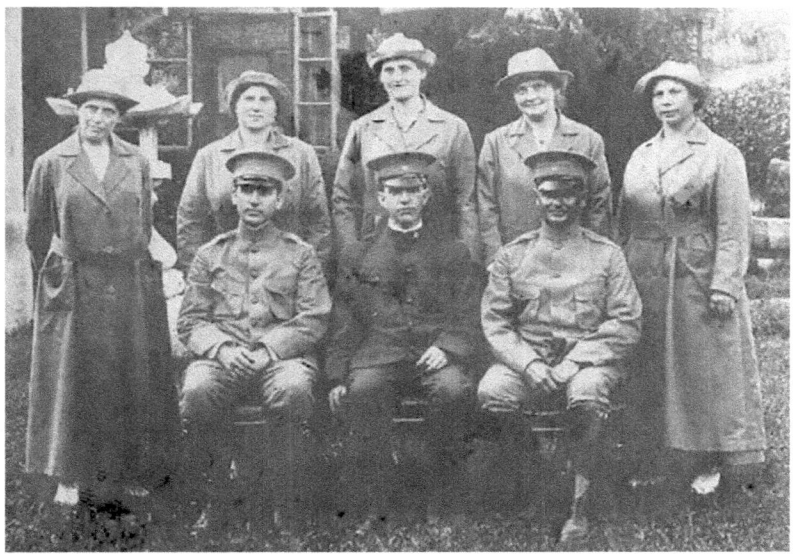

*Japan Chapter of the American Red Cross;
Delia is second from left in the back row*

We had just begun our much-needed vacation. We rested, read, played games, and swam in the Yellow Sea. We spent long sessions discussing the news that arrived from America about the war. It was quiet where we were, but we were apprehensive. Then a telegram arrived one day, saying that nurses and doctors were needed. Our whole camp was electrified. I could hardly sleep that night. The American Consul had requested that two of us come to Seoul. Caught up in the excitement, we all felt that it was a challenge worth meeting. We rushed to get to Seoul.

The United States had received a request to send an American Red Cross unit to Siberia as a medical unit for the Czech Legion, which had joined forces with the Allies[21] there. To get the unit quickly into the field, nurses and doctors already in Asia—primarily in China, Japan, and Korea—were being drawn upon. A group composed of three doctors and five nurses, myself included, was appointed by the American Consul

---

21. The main adversaries of World War I were the Allies, based on the Triple Entente of the United Kingdom, France, and Russia, and the Central Powers, based on the Triple Alliance between Germany, Austria-Hungary, and Italy.

in Korea to what was known as the Japan Chapter of the American Red Cross. We were led by Dr. R. B. Teusler,[22] who was director of St. Luke's Hospital in Tokyo, Japan.

Our group gathered in Seoul and made what preparations we could, given the limited time available. We were in a state of high excitement, as our great task was about to begin! We did not have time to wait for word from America with regard to supplies and regulation clothes, and since it was summer, khaki suits were made for all.

During the war, a force had been formed composed primarily of ethnic Czechs and some Slovaks, who were interested in achieving independence from the Austro-Hungarian Empire (the nation of Czechoslovakia did not yet exist). Many were conscripts who had been forced to join the German army but had deserted; others had been taken as prisoners of war by Russia. Organized and well-equipped by the Allies, they were called the Czech Legion and had been fighting mainly in Russia as a brigade within the Russian Army. They were to cross Siberia to Vladivostok and be transported back to Europe. They had asked for medical assistance, and so the American Red Cross Unit was formed in Asia to go to Siberia.

On August 7, 1918, dressed in khaki, our party arrived at the railway station at the South Gate in Seoul. Here, a large crowd of business and missionary friends, as well as Korean Christians, had gathered to see us off. We were given gifts of fruit and candy, and each of us was provided with a large box full of food for emergencies. What an inspiration it was to have these friends providing support. Good-byes said, we boarded the northbound train. Standing on the platform of our Pullman, we moved slowly out of the station but continued to wave to our farewell party as long as we could see them.

---

22. Rudolf Bolling Teusler (1876-1930) was born in Rome, Georgia and graduated from Virginia State University Medical School in 1894. After serving as a professor of medicine for some years, he went to Japan in 1900 as a missionary doctor with the American Episcopal Church. He started a medical clinic in the Tsukudajima section of Tokyo in 1901, and founded St. Luke's Hospital in the Akashi section of Tokyo in 1902. It is still in operation today as St. Luke's International Hospital.

Our patriotism ran high. When there was a catastrophe such as our beloved America at war, we didn't want to just read about it in the daily papers, we wanted to see and be a part of it. Now that we were on our way, we wondered what unforeseen adventures might lay ahead.

Our trip north through Korea was very comfortable; we traveled all the way in a first class train. We left Korea by crossing the marvelous American-made concrete bridge over the Yalu River. The scenery of the southern part of Manchuria was very much the same as Korea. If it were not for the Yalu River and the pig-tailed Chinese on the other side calling "hoo-hoo" to their mule teams, it would be difficult to tell where Korea left off and Manchuria began.

After we had journeyed for a day, I began to feel quite ill and had a splitting headache. Two days before I'd had a headache in Seoul, but figured that it was probably due to too much sun. All this excitement had happened in the middle of summer when the sun's rays are extremely hot. My face was flushed and my temperature elevated, so when we reached Antung, a town where we changed trains and had a three-hour layover, the party engaged a room at the hotel and put me to bed. The doctor diagnosed malaria and started me on huge doses of quinine. The party then gathered in the lobby to decide what to do with me. They considered sending me back, but after taking quinine and having a good sleep, my temperature dropped, the throbbing in my head ceased, and they allowed me to continue on. I was thankful that I was able to remain with the party.

Further north the country became quite flat. For miles and miles before we pulled into Changchun, we saw countless fields where the crops had failed due to drought. At several stations where we stopped, however, we saw great piles of sacks containing soy beans waiting for shipment.

Changchun

When we arrived in Changchun, Manchuria, on August 10th, we were expecting to go on to Harbin that night. Coming down from Harbin to meet us was an American Railroad Engineer,[23] who told us that we would have to remain in the hotel at Changchun until our American Red Cross train could be obtained and made ready. There were no accommodations available in the overcrowded, war-weary city of Harbin. Only the nurses stayed in Changchun, however; the three doctors went on to Harbin because they could live in the American officers' barracks.

To occupy our time we engaged a teacher and began to study the Russian language. We often became impatient because of the delay. We were anxious to be on our way and to start the work we had come to do. It seemed that everything moved slowly there, especially in war time. Patience was the lesson we had to learn; we were having our experience in "hurry up and wait."

Changchun was a large Chinese city with a great many buildings that were fairly modern. The streets were wide, but unpaved and dusty, and there were numerous open stands engaged in commerce. The shops, which were dark and dirty, had large signs with Chinese characters written vertically. We also saw some interesting ones written in English, like "Car Penter," "Watche Maker," and "Shoes and Boots Maker - Repairs Executed."

There was an upper-class wedding held at our hotel while we were there that we were able to see. The bridegroom was head of the Chinese bank in Manchuria. He wore a Prince Albert suit made from black silk, white cotton gloves, tan shoes with white rubber heels, and carried a high hat. The bride was a teacher at a girl's school. She wore a pink silk Chinese dress with a skirt, pink slippers and stockings, and a pink veil. The governor of Manchuria conducted the ceremony. He was a fine-looking Chinese man dressed in formal attire.

The couple bowed to each other three times, to the governor three times, and then signed the marriage certificate. The bridegroom gave the ring to his best man, who put it on the table. The maid of honor picked it up and gave it to the bride. They turned around and bowed

---

23. The author mentions both American Railroad Engineers and American officers of the Russian Railroad Service in this section; it is unclear if these are the same group or not.

to us two times, and we bowed in return. The bridegroom had two attendants; the bride was attended by two bridesmaids and four flower girls. The bride's students, wearing their pretty pajama suits, were present and sang. There was a big feast afterwards, which we did not attend.

We spent another interesting afternoon with a lieutenant from the American Railroad Engineers, who came and took us to a ball game. It was played by the Meji, a university team from Tokyo, and a local team of Changchun businessmen.

We often heard bugle calls and the tramping of feet. Day after day, thousands of Japanese and Chinese troops passed through the city.

A visit to a Lama temple afforded amusement and change. Since it was some distance away, we called a hack. What a contraption that was! It reminded us of a one-horse shay, but there were two horses, one horse in the fills and one running alongside. The horses, one gray and the other tan, were of medium height and scrawny. The harness was a precarious patched-up job of straps, old rope, and string. We sat in the back seat, and the driver, a blue-clad Chinaman with a long black queue, sat in the front. He cracked his whip and called "hoo-hoo" to his faithful horses as we clattered along the dusty, bumpy road. The unwatered streets were full of hacks that stirred up clouds of dust and made it almost impossible to see or breathe, necessitating a bath upon return.

Almost daily, sandstorms were whipped up by winds blowing across the Gobi desert. The trees on the side of the road looked sick. Their leaves were covered with layers of dust and curled back on their stems. Their branches seemed to lack the energy to make even the slightest movement. They hung listlessly down toward the earth with their burden of dust.

The temple was a small Chinese building with a tile roof turned up at the edges. It contained statues of many gods; each with a sacrificial dish containing food in front of it. Some of the gods were about eight feet tall. They were grotesque, with fat, ugly faces. Some were fierce looking and painted in gaudy colors, with a second set of eyes on their stomachs. Others, sitting on thrones, had beautiful yellow satin capes wrapped around their shoulders.

In back of the temple was an unusual Chinese graveyard. The coffins were made of heavy lumber and painted in bright colors. They had never been put in the ground, but stood row after row above the ground. In front of each was a pile of ashes where worshipers had built fires to make sacrifices for their departed loved ones. It was a colorful scene but we didn't linger. In spite of the sealed boxes, there were noisome emissions.

The welcome news finally arrived. A house had been obtained in Harbin for our American Red Cross Unit headquarters. We joyfully left Changchun and headed there, accompanied by an American lieutenant.

Harbin

In the early morning of August 30th we arrived in Harbin and went to our lodgings, a fairly comfortable place two blocks from the Red Cross office. We were glad to be out of the hotel and enjoyed getting these rooms settled for the Red Cross headquarters.

Harbin, situated at the junction of the Trans-Siberian and Southern railroads, was an important military point. All Allied forces were stationed there: Russian, Chinese, Japanese, Czech, English, French, Italian, Canadian, and American. It seemed as if every man on the street was a soldier in uniform.

On our first evening in Harbin we went to the YMCA at the American barracks to see a Charlie Chaplain movie. What an ovation we received from the soldiers. Clapping rhythmically and stomping in unison, they made us feel that, as American Red Cross nurses, we were welcome.

Here in Harbin we were told that some international change of policy had caused our delay. We were expecting to provide medical units for the 150,000-man Czech army, but we now learned that our mission was to go across Siberia and set up hospitals.

General Diedrichs,[24] reviewing his freshly equipped men one morning, was an inspiring figure. The martial music of a well-trained band

---

24. General Diedrichs was the commander of the Czech and Slovak forces in Siberia.

added to the occasion. With new uniforms and bright new guns, Czech soldiers poured in perfect order down the street in an almost endless line. Every soldier's eyes were turned toward their general as they passed by and saluted him. We were thrilled by the sight. As this well-trained, well-disciplined army marched along, one of our American soldiers turned to me and said, "My, but we are strengthened by these people."

We took our meals for several days in a Russian hotel where we learned to eat their cabbage soup. A Chinese cook was hired, and when a Korean boy showed up and asked to be with the people from Korea, we took him in as errand boy. Their poor command of the English language was the source of much amusement. The cook would say to the Korean boy, "Everyday go buy bread," to which the Korean boy would reply "No, you." The cook was told to get us a broom to which he replied, "You go catchy tiffin,[25] come back, I go catchy broom." Another time he said, "Now I go out catchy eggs, come back, half hour washy dishy."

Harbin was darkened by droves of flies that kept us busy with screens and swatters. The cook asked, "Why American lady no likey fly?" We told him that they carry germs and make people sick. "No worry, no worry," said the cook, "Fly no makey Russian lady sick." The cook went on to say, "Russian lady American lady no likey. American lady all time want clean, Russian lady no care."

There was a wood stove in the kitchen, so we told the cook to buy some wood. He said, "Come dark catchy wood." The next day our meals started to be served from our own kitchen. We never knew where the cook got the wood. The faithful devotion of the Chinese servant is remarkable; he will even steal for his master. We were glad to be out of hotels and to have home-cooked food.

While we waited for our train, we drove around the city seated in the back seat of a horse-drawn cab with a bearded Russian driver in the front. The horses had an arch over their heads, something I had never seen before except in pictures of Russia. We made use of our time by caring for some of the American residents there. We also helped do

---

25. Tiffin is a British colonial word for lunch or other light meal.

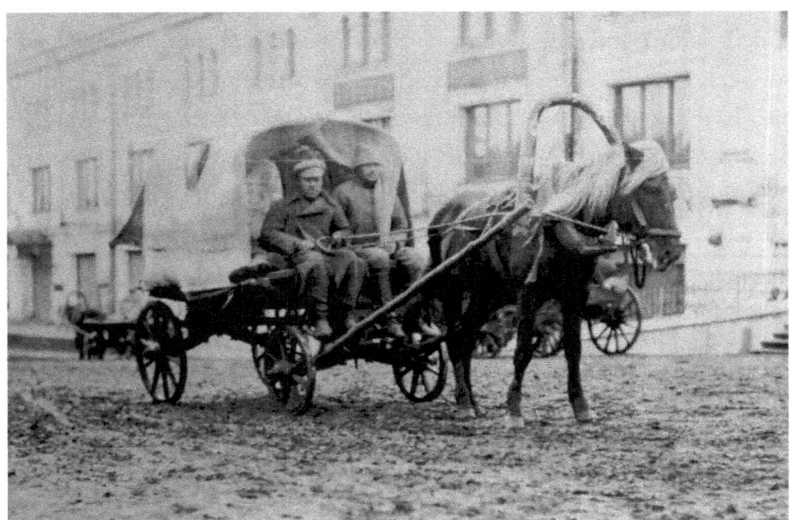
Russian horse-drawn cart

some buying for the Red Cross and provided ourselves with warmer clothes. Instructions had arrived from the American Red Cross headquarters in Washington, so we had regulation Red Cross uniforms and caps made. Later, when we found ourselves in the midst of a Siberian winter with temperatures sixty degrees below zero, we added fur coats to our equipment.

Harbin had aspects of Western and Eastern cultures. The new part was built around the railroad station. It had broad streets and buildings made from brick, stone, and concrete. Many Russian, Chinese, and Japanese shops were located in this area. In the Chinese section the streets were narrow, the shops small, and there was a large bazaar or open market where we found the money changers. Money changers interested me because they reminded me of the role they played in the Bible. They occupied rows of little tables on the street. Each man sat on a stool in back of a table which was about fifteen inches square. As I watched these men I wondered if money could be as muddled in biblical times as it was then in Siberia. All the cash had been hoarded away so only paper money remained. Not only rubles, but kopecks were in paper. From day to day, the value of the money changed, and we did not know on what day the money we held would be absolutely worthless. If we changed yen into rubles we lost by the exchange, yet on the same day, if we changed rubles into yen we also lost. Not only did we lose by the exchange, but if we held a large ruble bill we had to pay from two to twenty percent to have it changed into smaller bills.

We tried to make purchases in some shops where they wanted us to give the exact amount. They would rather lose a sale than take a large bill and give change. Servants refused to accept their wages unless it was in small bills. No one would take a torn bill, yet we were constantly having them palmed off on us. In addition to all of these problems, there was also a considerable amount of counterfeit currency in circulation.

Harbin was the center of a large agricultural district that was called "the granary of the East." The streets were poorly paved and filthy dirty. When it was dry the wind carried about clouds of dust, which made it almost impossible to see, and when it rained, one waded about in pools of water and mud in the streets. It was not unusual to see pigs running about the main streets of the city and weeds grew waist-high in the public parks and front yards.

Several months before we arrived in Harbin it was a scene of lawlessness and disorder. Homes were broken into constantly, and people shot in cold blood, sometimes for only a few rubles. People were continually being held up, opium smugglers abounded, and respectable people dared not venture out on the street after seven o'clock.

An American dentist admitted some Russians into his office at nine o'clock one morning, ostensibly to have their teeth examined. Instead, they pointed a revolver in his face. He was helpless because his own revolver lay on the table in the next room. They succeeded in getting away with sixty thousand rubles in money and jewelry. They were unmasked, so they easily could have been identified, but it was useless to try to prosecute because the police were in partnership with the thieves. When we called on the dentist who told us this story, his office door was chained; we had to prove who we were before he would open the door.

Order was not restored until the Chinese had instituted martial law.

Refugees

The huge number of refugees we encountered in Harbin presented a picture of misery that staggered the imagination. Some had fled homelands that had been devastated by war; others fled to escape enslavement by the Germans. They came there from different parts of Europe: Russia, Armenia, Bohemia, Assyria, and Serbia. There were English school teachers and governesses who had been employed in wealthy Russian homes. There were students from large universities in Russia. There were peasants as well as women and children from wealthy Russian families. When we read in the papers of the awful conditions of the refugees in Europe, it hardly seemed possible; brought face to face with it, we were forced to comprehend.

Some of the upper class refugees were able to find rooms, and some students found work. Among the refugees in Harbin were men and women who were prominent in their respective communities. They were the wrecks of once happy families: professors, school teachers, priests, and many wounded soldiers.

Among the most pathetic were those who came from Armenia and Serbia. They had been mutilated and driven from their homes by the militaristic armies of the Central Powers. Half-starved and emaciated, some were barefoot and clothed in little more than tattered rags. Large numbers of them had been driven from their quiet peasant homes, subjected to torture at the hands of the Turks, and cast homeless upon the world.

The first part of their escape from their own country was into Russia, and they had covered many hundreds of miles on foot. They were given limited help by the Russians and sent into Siberia. Among these people were a few who had once lived in America and were trying to return there with their families. They crossed the country in box cars; large numbers were living, eating, and sleeping in these small quarters.

Some who were sick came to the Red Cross home for treatment. One poor lady was brought in carrying a baby wrapped in rags. She had given birth in a congested box car while crossing Siberia. The baby

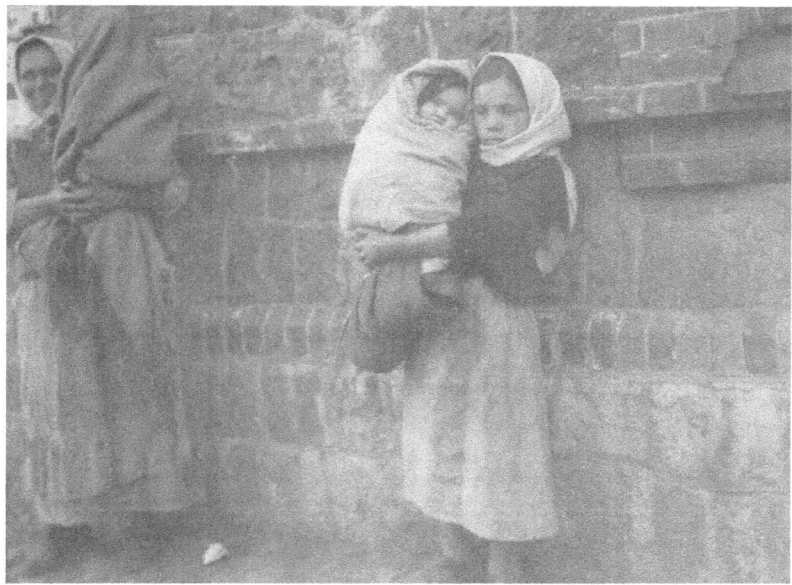

Russian hardship

was a cute mite, but had apparently never seen water or clothing. The poor mother told her sad and pitiful story in broken Russian, with many gesticulations. She stopped from time to time to cross herself, and to kiss the hand of the Red Cross nurse who cared for her. She said that her people had been driven from their homes and, weeping, she showed the scars on her face and body where she had been cut by the swords of the barbarous Turks. Her face was disfigured, but what was most cruel was that they had cut the tendons of her left hand, which hung uselessly from her wrist. She was given breakfast, a bath, and clean clothing. The pathetic little baby was also given a bath and dressed in warm clothing.

Later the same day, another lady appeared at the Red Cross home. Her left hand also hung helplessly and her body had been badly burned. She told a chilling story of how the cruel soldiers had put out the eyes of her infant daughter, right in front of her. Then when they seized her baby and threw it into the fire, she tried to save it and was badly burned. Such atrocities were unthinkable to us.

As some of these boxcars of refugees stood in the railway yard at Harbin, I decided to visit one. An Armenian girl of about eighteen took me there. She spoke a little English and clung to my hand as she led the way over the rails. She said many times how anxious she was to get to "Ameriek." When we reached the train we saw several small boys on the ground beside the car, making playthings out of wood and bits of things they found in the railroad yard. A woman took my hand as I stepped on a springboard and jumped into the box car. In the center of the car was a stove where dinner was being prepared. At both ends were stacks of wide bunks covered with pieces of carpet and matting; on these the people slept. There were only several women and two men in the car and some babies crawling on the bunks. The poor people in the car tried to smile, but their smiles had no spark. Their faces were lined and aged by what they had suffered during these hard war years. Lonely and homesick, they mostly just stood silently and stared with vacant eyes. At this time there were thought to be as many as ten thousand of these Serbian and Armenia refugees. As soon as the Red Cross learned the truth about their plight, they immediately arranged to feed, clothe, and shelter them. I felt guilty that my curiosity made me want to examine their distressed condition, but I was grateful for the opportunity to play a small part in the great humanitarian work of the American Red Cross.

We had one particularly enjoyable experience during our stay in Harbin; we attended a Russian-English class at the YMCA. There were several classes in English given throughout the week at the "Y." The class we attended was made up of about thirty men and women. Skill levels varied from those who had just started to learn to those who had studied for several years. There was also a social hour on Friday nights, attended by all of the classes, where Russian pastries and tea were served. The tea was served in glasses. When I inquired why they used glasses, a Russian man said it was to keep the hands warm. The Russians use sugar and lemon in their tea. If they do not have lemon they use a teaspoon of jam.

At these teas conversation was held in English and afterwards a talk would be given, also in English. For two weeks I was invited to give this talk, which I enjoyed very much. The class paid perfect attention as I told them stories in English. So eager were they to learn the language that they leaned forward to catch every word. I spoke slowly and distinctly to help them understand. For those who were beginners and had difficulty understanding, my stories were translated into Russian. It was most gratifying when I had them re-tell my story to me. I was sorry when I became too busy with my own work to continue.

American officers of the Russian Railroad Service were also stationed in Harbin. When one lieutenant became quite ill with pneumonia, we nurses went over to the officers' barracks to take care of him. He was placed in the hospital, which was a room at the end of the barracks. There were six beds and a red cross in the window; that was all. The workers in this so-called hospital were John, a Russian medical student, who gave medicine and treatments and took temperatures, and two Chinese boys who acted as orderlies.

We had nothing to work with. From the barracks washroom I obtained a wash basin, a sponge, and towels. The Chinese orderlies brought warm water in a ten-quart pail and set it on the floor for me to use. There was not even a screen. After bathing the man and making him comfortable, I had a carpenter come. He put up a frame across the end of the barracks. On this frame I tacked sheets so this very sick man could be in a room of his own.

While I took care of the lieutenant, I had my dinner and supper in the barracks' dining room, along with seventy-five American officers. There was a great deal of anxiety among the officers for this patient. Long before the nurses and doctor showed any sign of alarm, the colonel was sending cablegrams to his home. We did see the lieutenant through a very serious illness. At one point, we had very little hope. The doctors put his chance for recovery at one in a thousand. For days he talked in a restless delirium. He went through double pneumonia and pleurisy, and it was a long hard struggle. He finally recovered, however, and before we left Harbin he was sitting up in bed and eating his own food. How we rejoiced! As nurses, our real compensation was in seeing patients recover who were as sick as he had been.

All of the officers in the barracks seemed to appreciate what we had done; just before our Red Cross train pulled out of the station, we received lovely boxes of chocolates from the colonel, with compliments from the American engineers.

Chapter 10

OUR TRIP WEST ~ RUSSIAN UNREST ~ THANKSGIVING IN SIBERIA ~ TYPHUS HOSPITAL ~ RED CROSS HOSPITAL IN OMSK

Our Trip West

Time passes slowly in a war-ravaged country, where there were other high priority demands. Our Red Cross train was being equipped for us, but another sleeper was needed. One night, a train arrived with officers from the Russian Army onboard. Through persistent negotiation, our leader was able to acquire a second-class sleeper from them. He was anxious that we be as comfortable as possible on our long trip across Siberia. He stationed American soldiers to guard the train and came to alert us at two o'clock in the morning, telling us to be at the station in four hours with bags packed. In the mystic quiet of the early morning darkness, we were too excited to sleep, so we spent the rest of the night making preparations.

In the early morning frost before daylight, we went to the station. We found the car with an American flag and boarded it. After a dining car was attached and all preparations completed, we headed west out of Harbin at 11:30 a.m., on October 29, 1918: destination Siberia. We had the feeling that the task we had come for was about to begin at last, for we were now leaving Manchuria and entering Siberia.

Siberia is a legendary land of the north, known superficially to the world as a cruel, barren wasteland. It is thought to be a cold-storage dump for riffraff, malcontents, and dangerous revolutionaries.

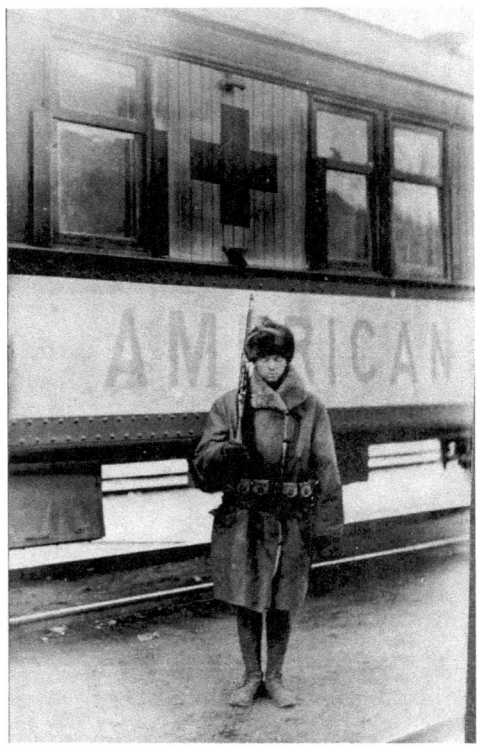

American Red Cross train car with guard

Although we were made very comfortable on our journey, everything we saw showed evidence of the disorder and confusion of the times. The beautiful Trans-Siberian cars were dirty and run-down, with bullet holes and broken glass showing that our car had been fired upon at some time. We beat dust out of the upholstery, washed the windows and woodwork in our cars, and sprinkled insect powder around our berth. The electric light system was out of commission, so we burned candles throughout our whole trip across the country. Most of the cars were in need of repairs and we traveled slowly because the railroad bed was in poor condition. Very little maintenance work had been done on the tracks because of the war, so the ride was rough and bumpy, and progress was slow.

Our Trip West ~ Russian Unrest ~ Thanksgiving in Siberia ~ Typhus Hospital ~ Red Cross Hospital in Omsk

The scenery along the way was superb and varied. We passed through great treeless expanses, known as steppes, and tundra on which herds of cattle, horses, and camels grazed. We saw low hills and high mountains in the distance. Then the scenery changed into beautiful wooded mountainsides covered by birch forests. The beauty of these white birch and evergreen forests set off by the snow-covered ground was beyond description. We also crossed many rivers, all of which had their outlet in the Arctic or Lake Baikal.

As we proceeded, we saw evidence everywhere of the destructiveness of war. At Olovyannaya we saw a bridge that the Bolsheviks had blown up. It was a massive iron structure that had stretched over the Onon River.[26] Our train passed slowly over a temporary structure built to replace it. Many buildings in towns and cities were burned and riddled with bullet holes, and there were many wounded soldiers in the streets. In close, smelly railway stations, refugees huddled together munching bits of black bread.

We arrived in Chita on the second of November. We had a few hours wait there, so we walked through the city and visited a beautiful Russian Orthodox Cathedral. The Russians appeared to us to be deeply religious people. There were icons in all the stations. Church doors were always open, and we visited a great many. One Sunday we saw a formal service. The Orthodox priests in their beautiful robes and stovepipe hats looked like prophets from the Bible, and there was an excellent men's choir. We usually visited churches on weekdays and saw the everyday concerns of the people at ceremonies such as marriages, baptisms, and funerals.

Babies were constantly being presented for baptism. Parents would hand their little naked baby to a priest and watch him plunge it three times into a large tub of tepid water. After one marriage ceremony, we watched a bride, who appeared to be about eight months pregnant, go over and kneel before her patron saint. We were surprised to see open caskets carried out and down the street at funerals, and found it hard to believe that communist agitators would blaspheme God by desecrating

---

26. Also called Lake Onon.

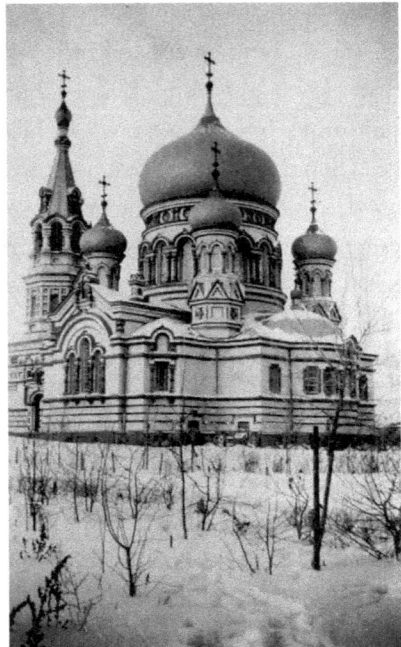
The Cathederal at Chita

altars upon which Christians had confessed their faith and dedicated their lives for centuries.

Chita was of particular interest to us because there were large prison camps located there. As our train stood on the tracks in the yard, another pulled up next to it. This train was carrying over a hundred German, Turkish, and Austrian prisoners. They had been prisoners for four years and knew nothing of their families and home. We told them that the German army was weakening, retreating ten miles a day, which was in the news at the time. They didn't believe it. "That couldn't happen to Germany," they said. One German prisoner spoke English very well. We talked to him for a while until one of the nurses gave him some newspapers with the latest news. He seemed very grateful for something to read. The prisoners were warmly clothed and told us that they had enough to eat. They could walk freely about the platform; there was no chance of escape because there was nowhere to go. You could look out over the flat frozen plains for a hundred miles and see no destination

Our Trip West ~ Russian Unrest ~ Thanksgiving in Siberia ~ Typhus Hospital ~ Red Cross Hospital in Omsk

worth running to. The Germans still seemed to retain their pride. While I was taking some snapshots, one German stepped back and said, "Let the Turks and Austrians be in the picture, not a German."

Continuing west from Chita we passed by forest-covered mountains until we came upon Lake Baikal. We were fascinated by the beautiful green color of the water. Picturesque mountains could be seen on the opposite side. It is a fairly large lake—about forty miles long and fifty miles wide—and is known to be the deepest freshwater lake in the world.

We visited the city of Baikal, which is located on the lake. As we approached it, we passed through a series of forty-one tunnels, the last of which been blown up by the Bolsheviks to obstruct the march of the Czech Legion across Siberia. It had since been repaired. There were many tunnels nearby that the Bolsheviks had intended to destroy. Had they succeeded, it would have taken at least three years to clear them out. The Bolsheviks were receiving financial aid from Germany for their revolutionary efforts, and the Czechs, deserters from the German army, were pushing their way across Siberia.

It was here at Lake Baikal that the Czech General Gajda[27] earned his reputation. It was said of him that he made no one his confidant. He carried out some of his greatest feats by deploying his men under sealed orders, which were to be opened only after reaching certain points. On this occasion he passed the word out among his men that if the Bolsheviks did not make it possible to pass through the tunnel soon, they would all starve to death. This news spread among the men, and was of great interest to embedded spies who relayed it to the Bolsheviks. Believing that they were in control of the situation, the Bolsheviks drew up in array for battle, including jubilant band music, and marched down on the Czechs on the battlefield. General Gajda was prepared. He had a decoy force deployed to meet the attack, which mounted a token resistance followed by a slow, tactical retreat. The Bolsheviks pursued them into a valley where the Czechs had prepared

---

27. Radola Gajda (1892-1948). His masterful Christmas Eve attack in 1918 took 20,000 prisoners and captured a huge amount of military hardware, earning him the nickname "The Siberian Tiger."

an ambush, attacking them from the hillsides. The result was a terrible defeat for the Bolsheviks. After this encounter the Czechs pushed on toward Vladivostok, clearing out Bolsheviks as they went, and gaining the respect of conservative Russians.

Irkutsk is a city situated on the east bank of the Angara River, the water of which is noticeably clear; as we stood on the bridge and looked down, we could easily see the bottom. While we were there, we visited the Museum of the Imperial Russian Geographical Society, which contained a great many interesting specimens and relics. Like so many other things in Siberia, the whole museum had a run-down and unkempt appearance. It too had been the victim of war. The outside of the building was completely marred by bullet holes. Inside we could see where bullets had cut through cases, destroying artifacts. A statue at the head of the stair was being repaired.

The Cathedral of the Virgin Kazan,[28] a church of the Russian Orthodox faith, was located in Irkutsk and we found time for a visit. It was a large modern building with five green domes. Inside, the walls were decorated with large paintings of saints and scenes from the Bible. There were massive gilt frames around the pictures and the walls were mounted with many brass candlestick holders and burning candles. The Russians were celebrating a holiday while we were there, and services were being held. Wearing a beautiful robe, the priest stood facing the altar with his back to the people. As he conducted the service, a chorus of rhythmical chanting accompanied him. There were no seats in the cathedral, so the people stood during the service. They crossed themselves many times and knelt from time to time, touching their heads to the floor.

As we walked about the street, we were surprised to find many buildings in complete ruin and the walls of schools, hospitals, and museums marred by bullet holes. The bridge across the river was also pitted with bullet holes, and a partially burnt boat stood near the bank. Rifles and

---

28. This cathedral stood on Kirov Square in central Irkutsk. It was considered a masterpiece of Russian architecture, but was closed and later torn down following the Russian Revolution.

Our Trip West ~ Russian Unrest ~ Thanksgiving in Siberia ~ Typhus Hospital ~ Red Cross Hospital in Omsk

shrapnel had left their marks everywhere. The whole city mirrored the destructive results of war and the revolution pushed by the Bolsheviks.

I was amazed to be riding on the great Trans-Siberian Railway, which I could remember learning about in grade school geography class. We traveled through a dull gray succession of days. It was often foggy and dark by three in the afternoon. The nights were long and cold; the sun didn't rise until ten o'clock the next morning. The ground was covered with snow that fell silently and persistently, transforming the landscape as far as the eye could see. The gold spires and colored cupolas of cathedrals stood out against a background of dazzling white. White birch trees stood proudly, looking as if they were part of the snow bank. The snow-covered steppes stretched out to an endless horizon.

At Tayga we took a branch line to Tomsk. There was some talk of organizing a thousand-bed hospital in this city. On the eighth of November we had a day to see the city. Tomsk was the most attractive city we had yet seen. It was well-known for its large university, which was the only one in Siberia. We visited markets, shops, and cathedrals. Droshky drivers here had exchanged their carriages for sleighs, so we had our first sleigh ride! We had seen them for days from our car window but had not been stopped long enough at any station to allow for a ride. The coachman looked like a mound of fur perched upon the driver's seat. We cuddled up in heavy blankets in the rear. The horses felt the invigorating air and ran along at a tremendous pace. There was exhilaration and a kind of joy in the air. The temperature had dropped below zero, and the dry sparkling atmosphere gave one a sense of well-being. Along the way we saw the humble homes of peasants. They had low thatched roofs and earthen floors. Families typically lived in a single room, often sharing the space with their farm animals whose bodies added warmth to meet the rigor of the long cold winters. When their load of heavy coats was removed, the Russian people appeared small, pale, and nervous.

Since it was decided not to open a hospital there we went on to Omsk, about five hundred miles to the west, where we arrived on the tenth of November. It was decided to locate a hospital here instead

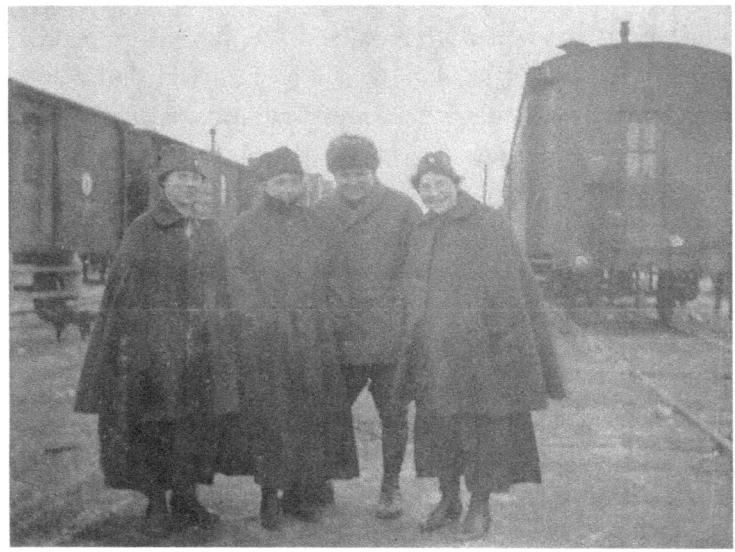

Life in the railroad yard; Delia is on the right

of in Tomsk. A building was obtained that was large enough for a thousand-bed hospital. Beautifully located, it was on the campus of an agriculture school. The building was being occupied by Cossacks, and it was two weeks before they could be evacuated.

We found it impossible to obtain accommodations in Omsk. The city was overcrowded, and people were living in boxcars, in boats frozen in the river, and in dugouts under the ground. There was no choice for us; we had to live in our cars at the railroad yards. Such was life on our journey; every day brought a new experience.

Our train stood on the track alongside other trains containing soldiers, refugees, and freight. At one point we were next to a French cavalry train. We could hear the horses snorting and stomping, day and night. Cows, pigs, and dogs ran freely about, and there was filth everywhere. We were thankful it was winter for we were at least free from dust and smells.

We could be quietly working in our compartment when, bump, we would suddenly get an awful jolt as our train was switched about. We were constantly switched here and there, and were continually finding ourselves in a new place, until it seemed we had occupied every spot in

Our Trip West ~ Russian Unrest ~ Thanksgiving in Siberia ~ Typhus Hospital ~ Red Cross Hospital in Omsk

the entire railroad yard. When we left the train, we often had to hunt for it when we returned. This wasn't fun in a Siberian snowstorm, when the temperature was below zero. One of the yardmaster's favorite stunts was to back us around during the night. One morning we found ourselves in a new place as usual, but to our surprise our car stood alone; we had been disconnected from our party. We remained disconnected for three days, until sufficient red tape had gone through and we could be coupled together again. In the meantime, we had to walk a quarter of a mile across the railroad yard for our meals.

Our train used candles for light, and water was hard to come by. Warm water would be brought into the aisles in a pail from the station. We would come with our basins and scramble for a portion, more than once getting left out. "Does someone want some warm dirty water?" was a common refrain. We were grateful for any opportunity to wash our hands before going to eat. What a luxury a hot bath in a tub would have been! Our first really cold morning, at 25 degrees below, we woke to find our car cold, the pipes frozen, and no water.

Although we spent a lot of time waiting, we always seemed to stay busy. We spent time sewing and knitting. We went out into the city to help with refugee work. We visited the Russian Orthodox Cathedrals, which we always found interesting. In the shops, shelves were often empty and supplies were hard to obtain.

Russian Unrest

Omsk was a capital city, and as such, was a place with many political complications. Many different groups were trying to control the government. Names like Kolchak, Kerensky, Trotsky, Stalin, and Lenin were often overheard. For us, it was a unique experience to be visiting a country that was in the midst of a revolution with all its rapidly changing conditions.

It was common knowledge that Russia had been in a bad state for quite some time. There was rebellion against the Tsar and his monarchical government, along with the generally unwholesome condition of the country. Wealthy Russians lived in extreme luxury while peasants struggled for a crust of bread. Any attempt to ameliorate the situation was met harshly by the police and could result in exile to Siberia; many political prisoners had already been sent there. Nonetheless, unrest had led to revolutionary ferment. The victory of Japan over Russia in the Russo-Japanese War had been an embarrassment for the Tsar and had contributed to the destabilization of his regime. A further scandalous incident had occurred during the war when a drunken Russian commander surrendered Port Arthur despite having a force that was well-supplied with food and ammunition.

In addition, controversy surrounded the Tsarina Alexandra, who had fallen under the influence of the mad monk Rasputin. She turned to him for spiritual and moral support after doctors were unable to successfully treat her son, Alexei, who had been born with hemophilia in 1904. Alexandra retired from public life soon after his birth to look after him, since the slightest bump or cut could kill him. Through some mysterious, hypnotic power, Rasputin kept Alexandra in a state of confusion, and through her he exerted a malignant influence over the Tsar as well. He had ministers he disliked removed at the drop of a word. The people looked upon him with fear, loathing, and contempt, until he was finally murdered in 1916.

The aristocracy and intelligentsia lived in terror as the spirit of revolution grew. Some, disguised in peasant clothes, fled from their homes. The Tsar was isolated and did not think too seriously of the unrest until it was too late. He still held to his belief in the divine right of kings. The final and fatal chaos was brought on by World War I. Revolutionary agitators took advantage of the state of confusion hastened by the war and started working in the open. By 1916, the entire machinery of the state was in a desperate muddle, as were the armed forces. The Tsarist army of fifteen million men was becoming exhausted. We were told that, while the people expected a revolution and knew it was inevitable, no one, neither the revolutionary leaders nor the Tsar himself, had understood how explosive the situation had become.

Our Trip West ~ Russian Unrest ~ Thanksgiving in Siberia ~ Typhus Hospital ~ Red Cross Hospital in Omsk

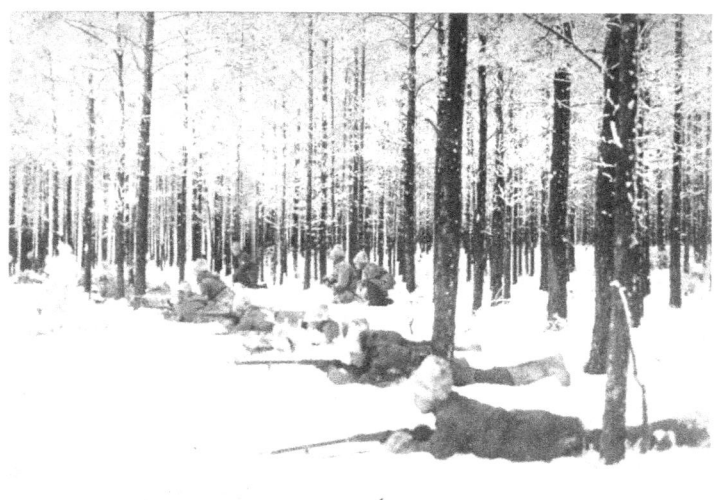

Soldiers in the snow

Prior to the October, 1917 revolution, Lenin was living in Switzerland, having been exiled from Russia. He made his plans from there, carrying on secret negotiations and making important concessions to Germany in exchange for aid and financial assistance. He had agents throughout Russia and had been able to form a formidable coalition from socialist parties, mutinous garrisons, and working-class people. Through relentless determination and persistence, he was able to overcome all other factions. By 1912, he was the indisputable leader of the Bolshevik Party, although he had no official title. The professional revolutionaries followed their party leaders without question. They thought of themselves as expendable. They had neither patriotism nor pity, and would lie, cheat, and murder to advance their cause. Their one faith was in the revolution, and on this subject they were fanatics. During the tumultuous year of 1917, Tsar Nicholas and his government were overthrown by the Bolsheviks.

In July, 1918, shocking news spread around the world. Late in the evening of July 16, Tsar Nicholas and his family were removed from Tobolsk, Siberia where they had been held captive and taken to

Yekaterinburg in the Ural Mountains. Here, the deposed Tsar Nicholas II; his wife Alexandra; their daughters the Grand Duchesses Olga, Tatiana, Marie, and Anastasia; and the Tsarevitch, Grand Duke Alexei, then only fourteen years of age, were all savagely murdered.

Yekaterinburg was only a short distance beyond Omsk, so the newspaper men in our party went ahead to see the building where this shockingly cruel and atrocious act took place. When the newsmen returned, one said to me, "Don't the Red Cross have guns?" When I told him that Red Cross workers do not carry guns, he said, "You people have no idea of the seriousness of the situation in this country." At this time we were warned not to use the word Bolshevik in our conversation.

One morning we awoke to learn that the city had been surrounded by soldiers with machine guns, and that we had come close to being fired on. The American consul advised us that if we heard fighting during the night to turn over and go back to sleep, for Americans were really quite safe. It was quite remarkable and comforting to know that American citizens were respected and protected in the land of revolution.

Thanksgiving in Siberia

Thanksgiving Day arrived while we were still in the railroad yard. Perhaps in Rome one does as the Romans do, but regardless of what country they are in, Americans do as Americans do. It was natural, therefore, that all the Americans in this bleak, frozen city of Omsk, Siberia, got together to celebrate one of our great national holidays. There was so little to work with, it seemed quite an impossible proposition at first. But when the consulate, the Red Cross, and the YMCA put their efforts together the result was a truly American festival.

The dinner was marvelous. We had roast turkey with all the trimmings, even cranberry sauce. Cranberries, by the way, were the only fresh fruit we had while in Siberia. For dessert, an English lady in our party had made a real plum pudding. The dinner was served in a large room at the YMCA clubhouse. We were surprised by the beauty of the decorations. There were evergreen clippings, American flags, Red Crosses, and YMCA triangles on the tables. There were places set for forty-two. Someone in the party had made bright little place cards with a strutting turkey and clever limericks on them. These were read between courses to everyone's great amusement. For tablecloths we used sheets, and no one seemed to mind that most of the knives and forks were steel and the dishes granite.

The food was good and it was made a happy affair because everyone maintained a beautiful Thanksgiving spirit. The conscious effort to produce a cheerful atmosphere could hardly be improved on. The conversation sparkled with stimulating wit. We were greatly favored by the Czech army, which sent a forty-piece band to provide music for the occasion. After we found our places, the band played "America." The American Consul General provided welcoming remarks, followed by the YMCA director who offered a Thanksgiving prayer and read the following nostalgic poem:

Thanksgiving Day
by Martha Haskell Clark

The little, wistful memories they woke with me to-day
Amid the pale-lit, primrose dawn that streaked the snow-clouds gray,
For when the first, wan light appeared upon my chamber wall
The little, wistful memories they waked me with their call.

Across my frost-ferned window-pane a hint of wood-smoke sweet,
Adown the hallways of my heart the tiny, stirring feet
Of dear and lost Thanksgiving Days, like children's ghosts astray
And little, wistful memories that woke with me today.

The little eager memories they crowded at my board,
They stilled the kindly stranger-voice that blessed our simple hoard
With low and half-heard whisperings in tones of other years,
That thrilled my trembling heartstrings through, and stung my eyes to tears.

The lighted room grows strangely dim, and through my lashes wet
I see in all its older cheer another table set;
Oh present, dear Thanksgiving joy, with heartache underscored,
And little, eager memories that crowd around the board!

The little, pleading memories, I heard them where they crept,
When warm upon the wide-armed hearth the dying fire-glow slept,
They slipped small fingers into mine, and watched, while dimmed
    and gray
There paled the last red embers of each past Thanksgiving Day.

Oh God, while here for present good I bring Thee grateful praise,
I thank Thee too for all the joy of old Thanksgiving Days,
For voices stilled, and faces gone, in living presence kept
By little, tender memories that sought me where they crept.

    The meal was most satisfying, and the after-dinner speeches were very good, so we all had a most enjoyable time. In addition to those of us from the American Red Cross, there were five YMCA men, the American Consul General, and several members of his staff. Other guests included the British Consul General and his staff of seven. There was also a group of British Red Cross workers we had met there: one man and three nurses. They were Quakers and conscientious objectors, but were here doing Red Cross work for their contribution to the war effort.
    That evening, in the early twilight, as one of the YMCA men was walking home with me, we had a narrow escape. A short distance from the club, a Russian soldier shouted at us. Fortunately, the YMCA man understood a little more Russian than I did—he was saying "Halt! Or I will fire!" We presented our passes, but it was too dark for the soldier to read them. Holding them up to his lit cigarette, he was finally able to make them out and handed them back. This absurd and perfunctory examination over, we went on unmolested.

The following Sunday we were invited to an English worship service of thanksgiving, observed by the 25th Battalion of the British Middlesex Regiment at their barracks.

Typhus Hospital

During this period there was an epidemic of typhus in the congested cities along the railroad. Typhus is an acute infectious disease, usually associated with overcrowding, inadequate sanitation, and poor hygiene. Such conditions favor the spread of lice, which serve as carriers and transmitters of the disease.

Here in Omsk, we were told that there were nine typhus hospitals scattered throughout the city. We visited one such hospital for refugees and found the patients in a most pitiable condition. The hospital was struggling—their drug supply was nearly exhausted and there was a shortage of beds, gowns, sheets, and blankets. There were ninety patients there with typhus or typhoid, and a few with relapsing fever. It was impossible to quarantine them and stop the spread of disease.

The building was a barracks—a one-story barn-like structure with concrete floors and whitewashed walls. In the center of the room were two rows of platforms built with boards. The platforms, which met at the center, had a slight incline toward the outer aisle and were covered with straw, like what would be used to bed a horse. The platforms were wide enough so that two rows of people could lie on them. The patients—men, women, and children—were placed with their heads toward the center and their feet toward the aisles. Their eyes were red and their faces were flushed and swollen. It was difficult for them to sleep and you could hear them muttering with delirium. Eyes would open occasionally to reveal a listless, helpless appeal. They were frightened, sick, and miserable, but clinging to life.

There seemed to be whole families lying together. I saw one poor suffering man and wife lying with their heads on the same pillow. In another place along the platform, I saw a poor wasted mother draw herself up on her elbow and try to do something for the comfort of

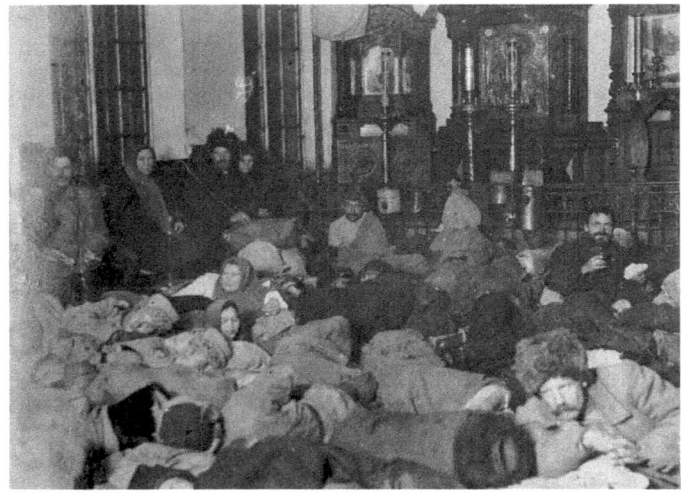

Typhus hopital

her three emaciated little children. The children lay listless, their eyes staring out of thin, pale faces. All they had to cover themselves with was their own clothing. Fortunately, the room was well-heated so they did not suffer from the cold in the subzero weather.

The Russian doctor in charge spoke English, which enabled the Red Cross to work with him effectively. The Russian nurses were strong women—hard-working and capable—and they did the best they could under trying conditions. They were devoted to the main tenets of nursing—to aid the sick and suffering to the best of their ability. They seemed well-organized, but the hospital was short of drugs, surgical dressings, and supplies. Many patients had been brought to the hospital lying on straw in the bottom of sleighs. They were taken first to an admission room, where they were put on a platform that lacked even straw. They remained there until the nurses and orderlies could admit them. In the admission or sterilizing room, as they called it, was a large bathtub and large sterilizer. When the patients were brought into this room, their clothes were removed and sterilized and their hair was clipped. Then they were put in the tub and scrubbed. Next, their sterilized clothes were put back on and they were sent to the next room on the straw platforms, which was called the clean room.

As unfortunate as the situation was, those who worked so faithfully with such meager resources deserved to be commended. Our hearts ached for the poor patients, however, and every one of us longed to give them clean beds in bright sunny wards. We could not do that, so we did what we could. When the hospital people saw that we were going to help, they cleaned and disinfected another room to which the overflow of patients could be transferred. The Red Cross furnished straw mattresses, pajamas, and large warm comforters for them, in addition to bandages and drugs for the almost empty stock rooms.

Later, when we went through the barracks to see the change, it was a paradise by comparison and we found the patients very grateful. We felt we had done very little, but the patients, although they could hardly lift their heads, looked up with wan smiles to say, "Thank you, thank you."

I went to bed that night hoping to rest, but I was too keyed up to relax. As I gradually began to quiet down, my mind kept returning to the events of the day and the scenes I had witnessed. I could not help but resent the unnecessary and useless war that brought with it so much needless human suffering.

Red Cross Hospital in Omsk

We finally obtained our hospital building and began moving in on the seventh of December. It was an agriculture school beautifully situated on a large estate on the Irtysh River, a branch of the Ob, just three miles from the city. We used the faculty house for our home and were very comfortable there. The school, a large three-story stone building, was not difficult to convert to a hospital. Plans called for a thousand beds, but while I was there only four hundred were available for use.

I was put in charge of a large surgical ward with fifty beds. We had patients that were Russian, Polish, and French, as well as Czechs, Tartars, and Hungarians. Communication could be difficult with so many different languages represented. One needed the gift of tongues. Occasionally, we saw the famous Russian Cossacks, crack troops that were well-trained and well-dressed. Most of our patients, however, were from the regular army and tended to be thin, dirty, poorly dressed, and covered with lice. Such was the state of the Russian army that, when the wounded came to the hospital, their overcoats were taken back to be given to other soldiers in the field.

To help us in our work, we were supplied with Czech soldiers as head men as well as German and Hungarian prisoners of war who served as orderlies. I directed these men with the little Russian and German I knew, often amusing them by using one word of Russian and two of German. It is surprising what one can do when there is no other choice. I made do somehow and, regardless of the language issues, the sick and wounded received good medical attention.

I was fortunate that the men working for me were good helpers. It was remarkable how well the prisoners worked for us, though not surprising, since they were told that any slackers would be sent back to the prison camps. Working for us they had plenty of good food, a warm place to live, and clean clothes. Most importantly, perhaps, they were treated with respect, so they preferred to stay with us and were very efficient workers.

Most of our patients were military casualties brought back from the Russian front, so we saw many simple gunshot wounds. We performed major surgeries of various kinds, and had numerous cases of frostbite requiring amputation. It was pathetic to see young men who had stood faithfully at their posts, often poorly clad, until they had become frostbitten. Many lost part or all of their toes and fingers. In the medical wards were the usual cases of pneumonia, malaria, and dysentery.

There was a global epidemic of influenza during the First World War and we did not escape it. We were all right until one day when a half-dozen infected French soldiers were brought in with it; several of our doctors and nurses contracted the disease soon thereafter. We received a further scare when typhus broke out among our patients, and at different times we had as many as twenty or thirty cases. These, of course, were sent to the typhus hospital in the city as soon as they were diagnosed. There were thousands of cases of typhus in Omsk, and many thousands in the other cities of Siberia as well.

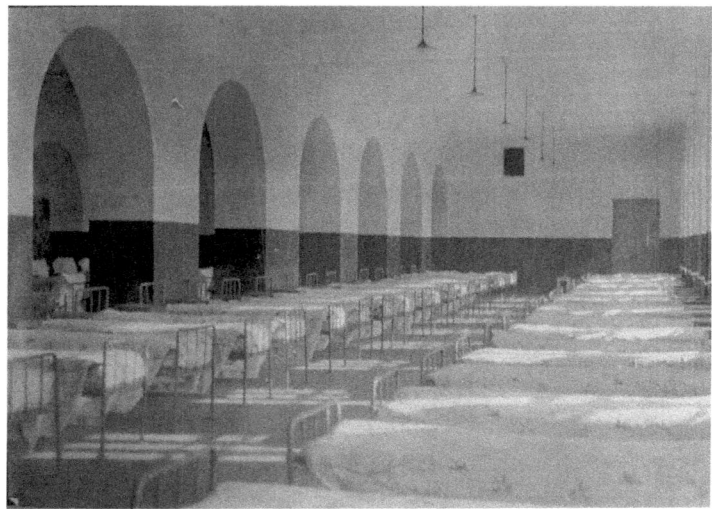

Red Cross Hospital in Omsk

The diet provided to patients in our hospital seemed strange to us, but since it followed the diet of the country, it suited them. Each patient received a chunk of black bread with tea for breakfast. If one man's chunk was not quite as large as his neighbor's we were sure to hear about it. Lunch was typically a greasy vegetable-beef soup, a dish of cereal, bread, and tea, while supper consisted of soup, bread, and tea. Each patient received half a pound of sugar a week. Milk and butter were given to the sickest patients. In the comfort bags at the head of their beds, patients could store away sugar lumps and bits of bread they did not eat; these they would carry home with them when they left the hospital. At times, when a group got together to play cards, I saw them gambling with their sugar lumps.

The wide road that led from the city to our hospital ran through a beautiful birch forest. When the ground was covered with snow and the trees, bushes, and fences were covered with frost, it was like a vision in fairyland. It was a beautiful trip into the city, but much too far for us to go conveniently, especially since we were unable to hire sleighs at the hospital. However, if we were not working too hard, we enjoyed walking into the city. Once we were there, we could always get a sleigh for the return trip.

For diversion we went for walks and sleigh rides, and attended concerts given by the English and Czechs. Occasionally, dances were held at the nurses' home. Many of our evenings were spent reading, writing, playing games, and singing. Every Sunday we had a religious service in our sitting room. One of the missionary doctors would conduct the service and, twice, the padre from the British barracks came out.

The cold was terrific, often reaching sixty degrees below zero. We had to learn to enter the cold gradually. There were two vestibules to pass through, and even with that, when we first stepped outside, we could hardly catch our breath and would have to cough a little before we could get adjusted. Pride in appearance went by the wayside, since we were wrapped up in enough clothing to look the size of mountains. We dressed in fur from head to foot and covered our heads and faces until only our eyes could be seen. I remember one day, when it was only twenty-five degrees below zero, we remarked how warm it seemed.

While we were in Omsk the political situation was in a precarious state. We were there when the government was overthrown and Admiral Kolchak,[29] leader of the anti-revolutionary forces, briefly became dictator of all Russia. It seemed like a quiet affair where we were, but Bolshevik disturbances were constantly arising, and at one point it appeared as though we might have to evacuate the hospital. For several days the city was heavily guarded and placed under strict martial law. All theatres and restaurants would be closed at eight o'clock, and no one was allowed on the street after nine without a pass. Everyone carried arms.

One day a Russian nurse asked me why we had come to their country to kill them. I assured her I had only come to serve, but by her attitude and conduct I could see she was a Bolshevik. There was no love among these people for Americans and many of these vodka-drinking Russians

---

29. Alexander Kolchak (1874-1920) was an admiral in the Imperial Russian Navy. He fought in both the Russo-Japanese War and World War I, and was briefly leader of a provisional Russian government in Siberia, commanding White Russian forces.

Our Trip West ~ Russian Unrest ~ Thanksgiving in Siberia ~ Typhus Hospital ~ Red Cross Hospital in Omsk

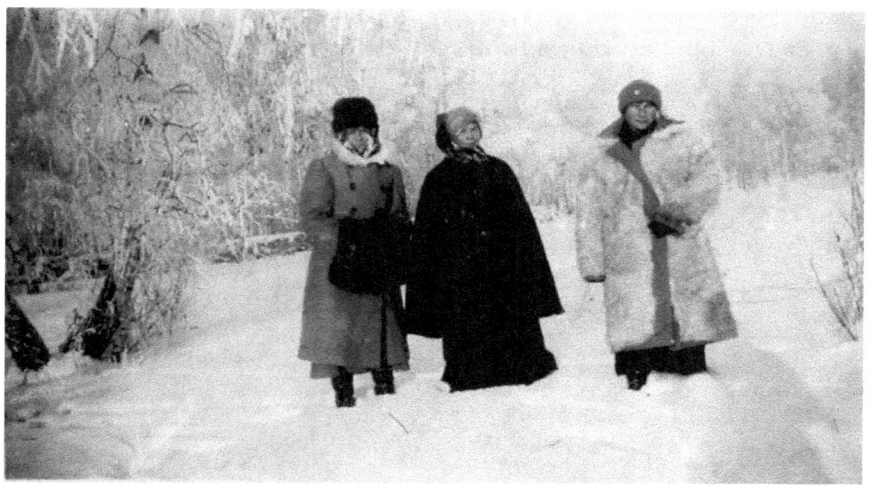

Dressing warmly for the Siberian winter; Delia is on the right

truly hated us. A few days before Christmas, 1918, a treasonous Russian guard set free about a hundred Bolshevik prisoners. In the struggle that followed, many men were killed. Because of the extreme shortages in the country, the soldiers stripped the clothing from the dead bodies. In the morning the frozen, naked corpses were found in grotesque shapes.

It was always a pleasure to work with the lovely materials that our American women had prepared for Red Cross hospitals. These supplies were packed neatly, well-made, and arrived in splendid condition. The Red Cross was a well-organized task force. It brought aid and comfort to people in their time of need and helped to maintain a friendly relationship between Russia and the United States.

The American Red Cross had large military hospitals in Petropavlovsk, Omsk, and Tyumen. They operated a tuberculosis hospital in Bukhedu, a typhus hospital in Petropavlovsk, and worked with refugees in Vladivostok, Irkutsk, Tomsk, Omsk, and Yekaterinburg. There were work rooms, baths, and supply rooms, and the Red Cross fed and clothed thousands of refugees. In addition, the Red Cross sent supplies to Czech and Russian hospitals at the front. They sent thousands of pairs of socks and sweaters to soldiers in the field, and clothing to the frontier for Russian soldiers returning from German prisons.

By the time I had been with the Red Cross for eight months, an armistice was signed and the war officially ended. Russian nurses had begun staffing our hospital, so I resigned my position. I was asked to join the medical staff on board a transport taking Czech soldiers back to Europe but declined, thinking it would be better to return to my mission work in Korea.

Chapter 11

OUR RETURN TRIP ACROSS SIBERIA ~ INDEPENDENCE MOVEMENT ~ AFTER THE WAR ~ SEVERANCE

Our Return Trip across Siberia

Our return party was led by a man from the YMCA, and included two nurses and a Czech soldier who acted as guard. As rough as we found the trip was going into Siberia, it was even worse coming out. We were given a fourth-class car with no comforts, just hard board seats. We piled extra blankets on and tried to use them for beds, but they were so hard that we couldn't sleep the first night. It reminded me of one of the soldiers who complained one day about the hard beds. He said, "It would be better to sleep on the ground. On the ground you can at least dig a hole for your hips." We slept on those boards for the entire journey across Siberia and they never did get any softer.

We nurses tacked up sheets at one end of the car to give us some privacy. We prepared our meals on a wood stove at the end of the car. One day, halfway across the country, our car was left standing on a siding. The mail train to which we were attached had gone on without us. The YMCA man located the station master and was able to use his permits and passes to prove that we were allowed to hitch our car to a mail train. After considerable discussion, we went on with the next one.

We visited the American Red Cross headquarters in Vladivostok, turned in our caps, and received honorable discharges. An American warship stationed in the harbor held a tea in our honor, after which we returned to Harbin. From Harbin we took a train south and headed back to Korea. After the awful bumping and jolting across Siberia, we were delighted to ride in the luxury of a modern railroad train.

After we had crossed the Yalu River and returned to Korea, we began to see things that puzzled us. As our train passed, we could see groups of white-robed Koreans congregating on the hillsides. As this was unusual, we wondered what could be going on. We soon discovered that we were jumping from the frying pan into the fire. We had come back to a troubled Korea. Not until we reached Pyongyang did we learn what had occurred in our absence.

Independence Movement - Korean Demonstration

According to the *Handbook of Korea*: "Japanese rule never succeeded in destroying the national spirit of the Korean people, but it was successful in suppressing Korean leadership and in weakening the latent capacity for assuming responsibility for governing the country."

Koreans are a peaceful people, but they have not always been able to enjoy peace. Situated as it is between China, Russia, and Japan, their land has often served as the battlefield for one country or another. Koreans have typically only fought in order to gain or preserve their freedom, not to acquire more territory by robbing their neighbors. They have tried for centuries to guard their boundaries and maintain autonomy and independence. Naturally, they chafed under Japanese rule. They had a chance to demonstrate their dissatisfaction to the world when President Woodrow Wilson advocated his policy of self-determination for all nations. Orderly and peaceful demonstrations were organized throughout the country, and a proclamation of independence was written, copied, and distributed. Meetings, processions, and demonstrations were planned in all the big cities.

Fortunately, the Koreans did not reveal their plans to the missionaries, since the Japanese would have loved to blame them for the independence movement. The real cause, of course, was the abolition of freedom of speech, freedom of the press, and freedom to travel outside of Korea, as well as the gradual loss of a great amount of land to the Japanese.

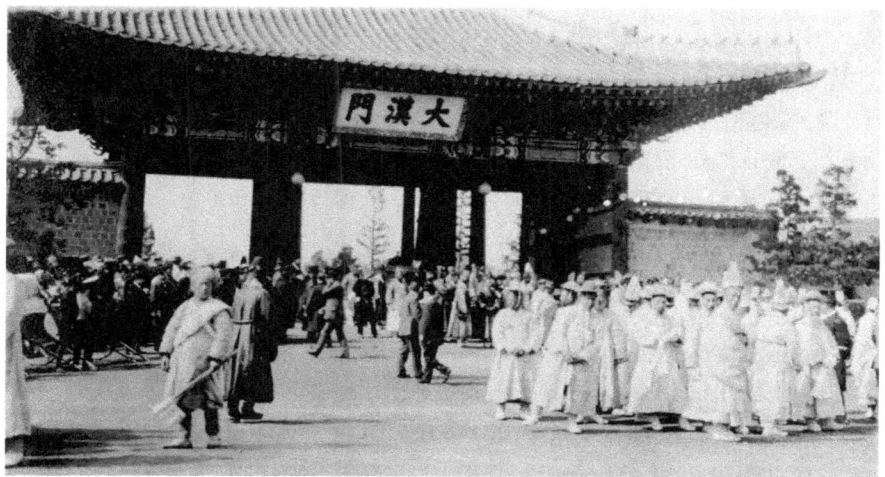

Korean street scene

The Koreans were held down in the past by leaders and overlords, and had never learned to hustle and do for themselves. They were gentle and trusting, and the shrewd Japanese found it easy to take advantage of them. Before the Koreans knew what had happened, the Japanese-owned Oriental Land Company had taken over farm after farm. The Koreans woke up to find that they no longer owned their land. They were knocked about, cheated out of wages, and had their houses and land taken away from them by the Japanese, who used tricks common to loan sharks all over the world.

The independence movement began on March 1, 1919. The proclamation of independence was signed by thirty-three Korean men, fifteen of whom were Christian, fifteen who were members of a native cult (the Ch'ondogyo), and three who were Buddhist. These men were immediately imprisoned by the Japanese.

Few believed that the Koreans were brave enough to face the Japanese and endure such great suffering for a cause they believed to be right. Nonetheless, at a given hour, millions of Koreans gathered in the streets throughout the country. Men and women, old and young, students and children, merchants and farmers, rich and poor: all were there. The presence of women was contrary to the age-old Korean custom of keeping them secluded. Casting aside their fear, everyone rushed about in the streets of the cities, towns, and villages. They threw their arms above their heads and shouted "Mansei, Mansei" — Long Live Korea! Forbidden Korean flags appeared everywhere.

It was a peaceful demonstration, and there were no acts of violence on the part of the Korean people. The same could not be said about the Japanese reaction, however. The police cut into crowds with swords and fire hooks, pushing, pulling, shoving, and dragging thousands to prisons, which were soon overflowing to an extent that was almost impossible to believe. Many cells were so full that people were in constant physical contact with each other, whether standing or lying down. In the summer, disease and vermin spread rapidly, and in winter many suffered frostbite in unheated prisons. Young women were subjected to particular abuse, often forced to undress for inspection. If they protested, they were struck. Medieval tortures were used to extract confessions from prisoners. Descriptions of such practices were constantly coming from the prisons: sharp objects were squeezed between fingers; people were strung up by their thumbs and beaten. Some were made to hold a chair or heavy board out at full length and were flogged if they let it sink the least bit. If they became exhausted and fell to the floor they were kicked and trampled on by the heavy shoes of the guards. If they fainted, cold water was thrown in their faces so the process could be repeated. Some were made to put their heads back as water was poured into their noses. Bodies were touched with lit cigarettes, prisoners were kept awake for long periods and compelled to stand in crouching positions until exhausted; the list goes on. The Korean people withstood this torture for as long as they could, but when they could stand it no longer, they confessed to whatever the Japanese wanted them to say.

Christians in particular were persecuted, which seriously affected mission work. Many of our Korean preachers, teachers, nurses, and doctors, as well as our personal helpers, landed in prison. Those who managed to avoid prison became fearful of attending church. Churches and Christian homes were burned; schools, hospitals, and homes were searched by the police; and in some rural areas, Christians were killed.

The meanness of life in the prisons did not dull the faith of the true Korean Christians. When the lights were turned off in the morning and on at night, it was a sign throughout all the cells that it was time for prayer. Christian preachers and teachers read the Bible and explained it to the other inmates. We were told that in room after room, non-Christians converted to Christianity.

It was fortunate for the Korean people that we were in the country. The Japanese suppressed the news so thoroughly that the world would have never known what was occurring otherwise. Even American missionaries in Japan believed that the stories emanating from Korea were greatly exaggerated. Our Mission Boards had instructed us that, as missionaries, we were not to take part in political questions; but when friends of prisoners continued to come back with news of such hideous cruelties, it seemed we could no longer stand quietly by.

At a meeting of representatives from various missions, we decided to take a stand—there would be "no neutrality to brutality." A letter was prepared and an appeal made to Japanese Christians, who immediately sent a delegation to Korea to observe the situation. To their horror, they found the stories to be true.

Faced with severe criticism, Japan began to institute reforms, though most were more apparent than real. One was to allow Koreans to study in their own language (the Japanese had planned from 1920 on to only allow Japanese to be taught in the schools). Another was to grant limited freedom of speech. Since every gathering was watched by police and spies, however, this was a reform in name only. In actual practice, if any free thought was expressed, the meeting was broken up at once. Even church services and prayer meetings were attended by spies. Some of the spies, not being Christians, could not understand such things as, "Thy Kingdom come," "The Army of the Lord," and "Onward Christian Soldiers." Many preachers were called before the authorities to account for their words.

Another so-called reform was freedom of the press. The Koreans had several newspapers, but the Japanese censored them each day before they were sent out. Sometimes whole editions were suppressed and publishers lost substantial revenues. After a few months of this, nearly all Korean papers had gone out of business. By the time I left the country in 1920, not a single paper was being printed in the Korean language by Koreans.

At their trials, prisoners were asked if the missionaries were behind the Independence Movement. Many of our Korean Christians told how they were tortured by the Japanese, who were trying to make the Koreans say that the missionaries were involved. On one occasion the English newspaper in Seoul, which was published by the occupation government, expressed how the Japanese felt about the missionaries. Its editorial read as follows:

> The stirring up of the minds of the Koreans is the sin of the American missionaries. This uprising is their work. There are a good many shallow-minded people among the missionaries, and they make the minds of the Koreans bad, and plant seeds of democracy. So the greater part of the 300,000 Christians does not like the union of Japan and Korea, but are awaiting an opportunity for freedom. These missionaries look at the present Korea as the old Korea. They think it proper to say anything they wish, if they only enter Christian schools. They take the statement of Wilson about the self-determination of nations and hide behind their religion, and stir up the people. The missionaries have tried to apply the free custom of other nations to these people who are not wholly civilized. From the part that even girl students in Christian schools have taken, it is very evident that this uprising has come from the missionaries.
>
> Behind this uprising we see the ghost-like appearance waving his wand. This ghost is really hateful, malicious, and fierce. Who is this ghost wearing the black clothes?—the missionaries.
>
> These missionaries who have come out to Korea, their wisdom, character and disposition is of the low trash of American Nation. They have sold themselves for the paltry sum of 300 yen a year, and crept out like reptiles on their bellies as far as Korea. There is nothing of good that can be said of their knowledge, character, and disposition. These messengers of God are only after money, and are sitting around in their homes with a full stomach. The bad things of the world are started from such trash as these. If we take all this into consideration these missionaries are all hated brutes.

We were told that less than a dozen Japanese lost their lives during the independence movement as a direct result of the uprising, whereas at least five thousand Koreans were killed and tens of thousands severely wounded—not to mention those flogged or otherwise tortured.

The Mansei Revolution, as it was sometimes called, seemed to end in failure. It did not achieve its immediate goal, except to the extent that the Koreans gained some self-respect. They also gained the respect of the foreigners who witnessed their heroic efforts to let the world know what was going on. However, Korea had to continue to endure privation and oppression at the hands of the Japanese militarists, who forcibly annexed Korea into their empire from 1910 to 1945. The Koreans were able to claim one particularly important accomplishment from the movement: the development of a government-in-exile. Delegates from all parts of Korea met in Seoul in April, 1919, and in the shadow of their persecutors, drew up a constitution and elected Syngman Rhee[30] as their President. It was not until July 24, 1948, however, that Dr. Rhee was officially inaugurated as President of South Korea. It took twenty-nine years of faithful and heroic service and the Korean crisis before the President-in-exile of a government-in-exile could take office as the first president of a free Korea. The *Handbook of Korea* called this the "first representative government in Korea's four thousand years of recorded history." We little realized at the time that Korea would soon be a battlefield once again.

After the War

To continue with the story of my return from Siberia: After getting off the train at the station nearest to Haeju, I was obliged to spend the night in a Japanese Inn in order to wait for the morning bus. The usual small charcoal fire provided warmth to the room. Since this was a familiar sight, I did not give it a passing thought. To my surprise, when I awoke

---

30. Syngman Rhee (1875-1965), also known as Yi Seungman, was president of South Korea from 1948-1960, presiding during the period of the Korean War. He was a Christian and died in exile in Honolulu.

the next morning I was deathly ill from carbon monoxide poisoning. By the time I reached Haeju, I was too sick to hold up my head.

As the days passed I gradually threw off the poison, but found it difficult to adjust to the resumption of my old life. I began to understand why soldiers returning from war are restless and uneasy and find it difficult to adjust. Back in Haeju, I found the empty space I had left there was strange and different. I no longer fit into it. Who has not had the experience of a discontented mind? I found myself starting to drag a little. My shoulders ached and I was unable to start off the day with a runner's spurt. I felt lost, like it was impossible to choose which loose ends needed to be picked up. It was time for a fresh start, a change of scene, and a new environment to stimulate my energy and make me feel like new again.

On several occasions I had been asked to join the staff at Severance Hospital in Seoul. This time, however, the request was a little more urgent. It was difficult to make the decision to leave Haeju for Seoul, but when I finally did, I found I had gained a richer and fuller experience. My appointment was made by the Bishop, and I would be the first Methodist nurse to join the newly established Union Hospital of Severance.[31]

Severance Hospital had been around for a long time. They had a medical school that trained young Korean men in Western medicine to become doctors and a large clinic that treated two hundred patients daily. They also had a one-hundred bed hospital. The hospital was originally built for thirty-five beds, but the work had grown so rapidly that basement rooms had been made into free wards. There was also a nursing school that could accommodate thirty-five student nurses. While I was at Severance Hospital I was delighted to be able to work with two nurses who had been with me in Siberia.

---

31. Severance Hospital is still in existence and is now associated with the Yonsei University Health System in Seoul. Founded in 1885, it was the first Western-style hospital in Korea.

Severance

Medical Missions were the wedge that opened Korea to Christianity. It was in 1884 that Dr. Allen,[32] a missionary to China, entered Korea. This was during a period when the people were very hostile toward foreigners, and there was a political struggle going on between progressive and conservative parties. During a coup attempt, a member of the royal family was injured and would have died if not for the prompt attention of Dr. Allen. As a result of this incident he became a confidant of the King, who offered him a building to establish a hospital. That King showed favor to the missionaries as long as he remained on the throne.

In 1905, the hospital was turned over to the Presbyterian Mission. A medical college was added in 1912, thanks to a generous gift from Louis H. Severance of Cleveland, Ohio, who was a captain of business and industry and one of Cleveland's foremost philanthropists. The institution then became known as the Severance Union Medical College and Hospital. When I joined the staff, Dr. O. R. Avison[33] was in charge. Medical missions represent Christianity in action, and I am grateful for the five years I had the privilege of being connected with this phase of the work.

Miss Esteb was in charge of the training school, Miss Reiner the main hospital, and I the college building and dispensary. Our division of labor worked well until Miss Reiner had to leave in April due to health considerations.

---

32. Horace Newton Allen (1858-1932) served as Presbyterian missionary and doctor in China and Korea. His connections to the Korean government led to his becoming involved in diplomatic relationships between the U.S. and Korea in the late nineteenth and early twentieth centuries. He also translated Korean literature into English and wrote about Korean foreign relations.

33. Oliver R. Avison (1860-1956) was a Canadian physician who served as a Presbyterian medical missionary in Korea. He was instrumental in stopping a Korean cholera epidemic through education and Western medical treatment. A speech he gave in New York in 1900 caught the attention of Cleveland industrialist Louis H. Severance. With funding from Severance, he expanded the hospital and developed the medical school. He has been called "the father of modern medicine and medical education in Korea."

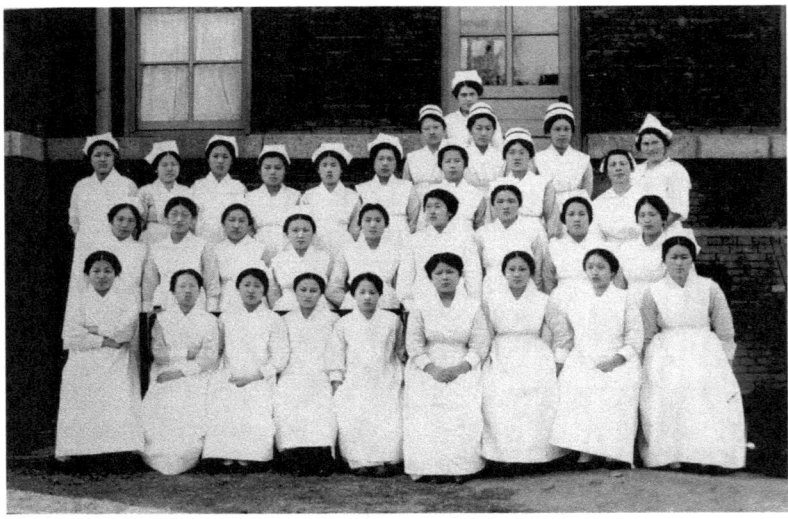
Severance Hospital nursing students; Delia is standing in the upper right

Again the work was divided, this time in two. Miss Esteb took responsibility for the training school, hospital, and Korean nurses' home, and I did the same for the dispensary, isolation building, and foreign nurses' home.

All the food for Western patients was prepared in our home. Sometimes, Western patients would stay in our home when the hospital's private rooms were full. I had to supervise our Korean cook as he prepared and served as many as six or seven trays for each meal from our kitchen.

I worked with all the Korean nurses as they came, seven at a time, to the dispensary for their two months of in-clinic training. These nurses prepared dressings, sterilized the supplies, and assisted the doctors in the treatment of patients. I found special pleasure in my work during this year and felt I had a closer fellowship with the nurses because I was able to teach my classes without an interpreter.

The Korean nurses here were better educated and more accustomed to Western people. They enjoyed their work and the instruction they were given. They entered into their nurse training with serious interest. We were challenged to set and achieve higher goals here because we could see concrete results from our efforts. It is significant that I could share in the training of these girls at that particular time. We little dreamed then of another worldwide conflict or a time when Westerners would be forced to leave the country. How fortunate for Korea that well-trained doctors, nurses, and hospitals were there to care for their sick and injured.

Due to political considerations, no graduation ceremony was held for nurses in 1919, so the following spring, the 1919 and 1920 classes graduated together. It was an impressive sight: sixteen wonderful girls standing up to receive diplomas. My heart swelled with a special pride because the top student in the graduating class was a girl whose training had begun with me in Haeju. There are many difficulties in nursing work, which help make us strong, but there are rewards as well. I was privileged to sign that girl's diploma and pin on her graduation pin before I left for home. God is good, for of sixteen graduating nurses, nine went up for their Government examinations. As I watched them and thought of my own training days, I was reminded how very human these girls were. They were so excited and keyed up before they went, and when it was over and word came that they had all passed—oh, there was such singing, shouting, and joy!

Chapter 12

NEW GOVERNOR-GENERAL ~ CHOLERA ~ ENDING

New Governor-General

A new Governor-General from Japan was sent to Seoul to become the new chief executive of Korea. It was understood that his would be a more liberal administration. There was a great deal of commotion in the streets and a large crowd gathered on the sidewalks to watch as dignitaries welcomed him and escorted him to his new home. Soldiers stood at attention ten feet apart along the route of travel from the South Gate Railway station to the government buildings. Our hospital, just across the road, gave us a good vantage point from which we could observe the proceedings. We watched as city police shoved the last bicycles and oxcarts out of the way, and two patrol cars arrived to block off the streets.

Thousands of people lined the street. The Koreans, all in white, stood alongside Japanese in colorful kimonos. There was tension in the air, and a feeling of apprehension. Although it was obscured from our vision, we could hear a train puffing into the station. The crowd booed and roared. Suddenly, we heard an explosion. Instinctively, people in the crowd tried to run, but there was no room. The mob became a surging mass, everyone pushing, shoving, shouldering, and veering to the right and left. Faces of the people showed panic and fear. There were Korean faces, Japanese faces, and Chinese faces. Anguish and horror was written on all. I shall never forget the wild eyes of the people in that human stampede.

As people turned and tried to get away from the station, the crowd became denser. Korean mothers frantically tried to protect the babies strapped to their backs. The hard hats of the Korean men toppled tipsily to one side. Driven ahead by the fear of the unknown behind, the people rushed, lunged, and pushed ahead. Bodies pressed against bodies, the sea of human beings becoming as one.

Amidst the panic, I marveled at the discipline of the Japanese soldiers who remained rooted at their positions.

"Why don't they help? Why don't they check the mob?" I asked my companion.

"They haven't been given an order to move," was the reply.

It seemed like odd behavior, but it spoke well for the Japanese soldiers' military training and discipline.

When and how the crowd dispersed I never knew, for there was no longer time to watch the street scene. Many at the station had been injured and were being carried on stretchers into the clinic, so our services were needed. When all the available stretchers and dressing tables had been filled, we placed the remaining injured in rows on the floor of the corridor. Taking the worst injuries first, we helped the doctors disinfect, suture, and dress and bandage wounds.

Among the injured was a young American couple. They knew nothing about the new Governor-General, and little dreamed of the chaos they would encounter during their visit to Seoul. Fortunately, their injuries were slight; we treated them and sent them on their way.

Who instigated the trouble I never found out, but it seemed apparent that Japanese rule was still not welcome in Korea.

Cholera

An epidemic of cholera broke out in 1919, causing consternation and panic in Seoul. When an epidemic begins, it usually will not end until there is a frost. The bacterium that causes cholera can live in salt water, so the disease is apt to travel from port to port.

During the epidemic there were hundreds of cases. Many patients crawled to our hospital seeking help. My heart ached for these poor creatures and I longed to take them in and care for them. Unfortunately, the Japanese government would not allow our hospital to handle these cases; they were carried off to the Government Contagious hospital.

A rumor spread that the police were receiving seventy-five yen for every case they found and turned in. Koreans were so frightened that no one dared to lie down if he became ill. It disturbed the Koreans very much, because although they didn't mind people with cholera being taken to the isolation hospital, they objected to the practice of taking people there for any illness whatsoever.

One day, a man coming into the city was seized on the street. He was on a street car and noticed that it was passing his stop so he hurriedly jumped from the car. A policeman, who was also on the car, suspected a guilty conscience and chased after the man and arrested him. When he asked why he was arrested, the man was told that it was because he was a cholera patient. The policeman said that he had seen so many cases that he could tell when people had the disease by their eyes. The man refused to go to the police station until it was proved that he really was a cholera patient. Because he resisted, the policeman beat him. This infuriated a crowd that had begun to gather and they threatened the policeman. The man insisted on going to the hospital, so the policeman brought him to Severance. The crowd followed, increasing in size until about five hundred were gathered at our door. The policeman and his prisoner were escorted into the vestibule and the doors barred to hold back the crowd. The policeman phoned for help with the disorderly mob. About twenty officers responded and soon the street in front of the hospital was lined with mounted police. Little by little, they broke up the crowd and sent them away. Once the crowd was dispersed, they took the arrested man to the police station, where he was eventually released—but not before he was pronounced a cholera carrier.

Our hospital played an active part in a campaign of prevention, setting up a free clinic for the dispensation of anti-choler vaccine. We maintained a twenty-four hour clinic in the railway station across the street from the hospital. This provided a real service, since Japanese regulations were so strict that no one was allowed to buy a ticket or ride on the trains without having first received the vaccine.

In previous outbreaks of the disease in Korea, people would have carved ugly faces onto posts and set them along the roadside with an inscription like: "This is the General who is after the Cholera devils." That is what they would have trusted to frighten the disease devils away!

Shortly after the cholera epidemic, I found myself in the midst of another. I was asked to spend the night with a very ill Salvation Army Colonel. I nursed him through a restless night of burning fever. In the morning I gave him a soothing bath and was startled to find that he was covered from head to foot with smallpox. During this mild epidemic, Korean patients were taken to the Government Contagious Hospital, but Western patients were brought to our pavilion. In all, I personally came into direct contact with twenty-one cases of smallpox.

For years the Korean people considered smallpox to be a disease of childhood. Many children were not given a name until they had survived the disease. When I first arrived in the country I noticed many badly pitted faces. The disease was gradually being contained by the Japanese government, however, which enforced a strict vaccination program. The smallpox vaccine had previously been unknown in Korea. One of the early reforms instituted by the Japanese after they took over the country, apart from cutting off men's top-knots, was compulsory vaccination. Japanese soldiers, in full dress uniform and with swords at their sides, went from house to house to vaccinate the people. This proved a great blessing, for it nearly stamped out smallpox in Korea.

In our hospital we treated all the common medical diseases such as typhoid fever, pneumonia, nephritis, malaria, dysentery, cholera, smallpox, and trachoma. While I was there I saw cases of tuberculosis and venereal disease that were more severe than any I had previously seen.

One day, an anxious, agitated man appeared at the hospital. He seemed as if he were under great mental strain. His face was lined, the pupils of his eyes were tiny, and the pigment of his skin was unnaturally yellow.

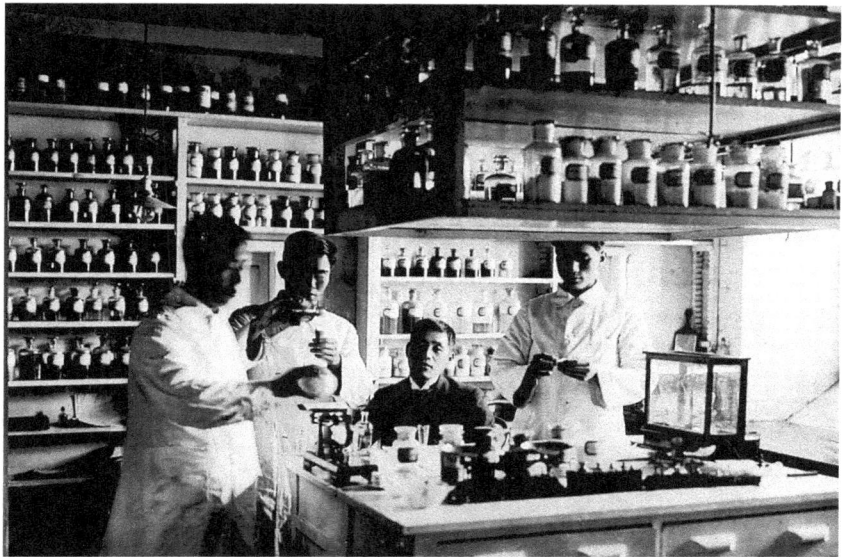

Severance Hospital dispensary

These symptoms told us at once that he was a drug addict. He asked for morphine. When the doctor refused to give it to him, he begged and begged. The doctor tried to explain to him that one dose would do no good and that he lacked the means to cure addiction, so he could not give out morphine. The man paused, but then dropped to the floor on his knees with a helpless expression, put his hands to his head, and began to rock back and forth. His face was contorted in agony, and he pleaded for relief. After a while, one of the hospital attendants helped him to his feet and persuaded him to move on.

We took care of all diseases common to women. I felt a special sympathy for women who came to the hospital seeking treatment for sterility. It was such a curse to be unable to produce a son in Korean culture. Many a poor wife saw her position superseded by a concubine. One young woman came to the hospital to be treated for an incarcerated uterus. She said to us one day, "As for my baby house (uterus) it is alright, only 'Naug' is the trouble." She would let the old Korean doctor stick his long needle in to try and kill the "green eye." Who wouldn't want to get rid of something that caused so much discomfort?

If I were asked what primary afflictions were common to Koreans, I would say indigestion and worms. This was because of the foods they ate and poor sanitation. Hardly a stool was examined in which we did not find worms: whip worms, round worms, tape worms, and hook worms. Giving a routine treatment for worms would be considered old-fashioned at home, where they are uncommon. In Korea, however, we were continually pulling protruding and wriggling worms from the noses and rectums of patients. Patients would even vomit worms. When hundreds of people got their water from a common spring, washed their clothes and vegetables at the same place, and fertilized their gardens with human waste, it was small wonder that the soil and water were polluted.

The most pathetic and certainly unnecessary medical cases we saw occurred as a result of flogging. The Japanese government believed in corporal punishment and for certain crimes ordered a number of strokes to be given. The man to be flogged was stripped and laid face down on the ground or tied to a bench, making it impossible for him to move. The flogger would strike him on the buttocks with a flexible paddle for as many counts as ordered: twenty, thirty, or sixty strokes. The cruelest order was for thirty strokes applied for three consecutive days. Adding more strokes to the already sore and inflamed flesh caused the buttocks to become lacerated and infected. The traumatic injuries induced by this fiendish torture often required surgical care. The muscles of the buttocks in many cases broke down and became suppurated. Surgeons had to make a cross incision in these inflamed areas to establish drainage, followed by a daily change of dressing. Such wounds took a long time to heal, and the patients were left unable to sit for many weeks.

Missionary doctors tackled problems of Asian diseases unknown in America, such as scrub typhus, Japanese encephalitis, hemorrhagic fever, and sprue (celiac disease). Unfortunately, the day-to-day grind of treating common diseases such as ulcers, boils, ringworm, and croup did not always allow doctors the stimulation of conquering new and unknown diseases.

Dr. Irving Ludlow,[34] head of the medical school, made a special study of liver abscesses while in Seoul and became a world authority. Stimulated by his interest in the condition, I wondered how many cases we might have in the hospital. One day I went through the private rooms and various wards. On that one day I found seven cases. This was especially interesting in light of the fact that many doctors at home had never seen a liver abscess at all.

Our surgical ward was also a busy place. We operated on eyes, ears, noses and throats. We performed amputations and many abdominal surgeries. We also did a great deal of plastic surgery.

Ending

"Ideals are like the stars, we never reach them, but like the mariners of the sea, we chart our course by them."

A sunny day, it is late enough in winter to have the feel of spring. The bare trees and shrubs still look dead, but in reality they are pregnant with life. The buds are perceptibly swelling. In a few short weeks the miracle of leaves and multi-colored flowers will emerge. It is spring; everything is alive as are we. How wonderful this spring fever is: to be happy, to be alive. Are we not in the Master's hands? He told us in his Word that the birds that He feeds do not want, that the flowers He clothes with exquisite beauty do not want. Our part is to seek and establish God's Kingdom on Earth. The Kingdom which we seek is real, and our Heavenly Father plans for us to attain it. Jesus expressed it this way: "Fear not, little flock, it is your Father's good pleasure to give you the Kingdom." Even though there are few of us, we need not worry. If God has heard the prayers that have ascended to Heaven on behalf of Korea, He is working things out to that end. Each missionary

---

34. Alfred Irving Ludlow (1876-1961) served as a physician and protestant missionary in Seoul from 1912-1938. See also the article on page 167.

can do only a small part. Daily work and prayer in one's lifetime yields so little progress, but to me it is enough to have been a part. I always think of a pyramid: each worker adds a stone. Someday perhaps some outstanding person will lay the top stone of the pyramid. His name may go down in shining lights as having brought Christianity to Korea. Who this person will be we now have no idea. But I do know that without my little stone in the pyramid this person would never have reached the top. The stones consciously placed there by all the people who have worked in Korea are of equal importance.

"To my virtues, be most kind, to my faults, a little blind." Those were indeed interesting times.

Appendix I – Miscellaneous Notes

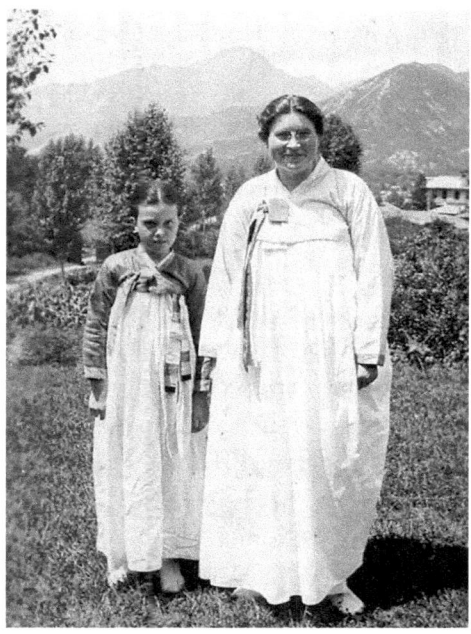

Delia and a young friend, in traditional Korean dress

Appearing in the *Cleveland Press*, Jan. 1, 1951 ("Korean War Ruins Hospital Built by Clevelanders" by Ken Marino) - the following:

> Dr. Ludlow has just received a letter dated Dec. 6, 1950 from his successor at the hospital, Dr. Y. S. Lee, who returned to Seoul after three months as a refugee in the south. He wrote that "bombs have destroyed 60% of the hospital buildings and the Reds have stolen or burned 90% of the equipment."
>
> "Just three walls of the main building remain," the letter said, "and the old three-story hospital, the nurses' home, the staff residences and the Severance-Prentiss Wing, the dental building, the tubercular isolation ward—all are demolished."
>
> Dr. Ludlow recalled today that the hospital was situated only 300 feet from the Seoul railroad station, on South Gate St., just outside the old city. He said, "The letter doesn't hazard a guess at whether they actually shelled the hospital buildings or were aiming at the railroad station,

but the destruction is just as final. The loss of the buildings, although sad enough, is trivial when one thinks of the number who must have died or been hurt in the shelling. The hospital was always crowded with patients. The doctors, nurses and technicians lived on the grounds. This is a sad blow." ....

"The North Koreans tried to hunt down and liquidate all of the nine hundred doctors the medical school had graduated and the five hundred nurses trained in the nurse's school there since the founding of the institution. Apparently, intelligent people are regarded as dangerous by the Reds."

ᛰ   ᛰ   ᛰ

After thirty-five years, there are three hundred thousand Christians praying and studying the Bible in Korea—thanks to missionaries. If you ever saw, as I did, hard, heathen faces transformed into bright, happy ones, you could never doubt the life-altering power of Christianity. When a Korean becomes a Christian he becomes a proselytizer and spreads the word to others about the "Jesus doctrine."

A family of Presbyterian missionaries in Korea once took a Korean girl back to America to give her a chance to study in our schools. Crossing the country by train, she aroused the interest of some passengers who engaged her in conversation. In the course of these discussions she asked one man if he was a Christian. When he said no she reported back to the missionary and suggested that he speak to the man. Most American preachers are not in the habit of speaking to fellow passengers in a train about their soul's salvation, but this missionary didn't want the little Korean girl to lose her faith in him, so he went back and spoke to the man. He told him that the Korean girl was concerned about him because he was a heathen.

"Am I a heathen?" the man asked.

"Yes," replied the missionary. "You are not a Christian because you do not believe in the Lord Jesus; therefore you must be a heathen."

This idea struck the man so forcibly that, after returning to his home in San Francisco, he wrote to the missionary and asked him to tell the Korean girl that he, his wife, and his whole family had joined the Presbyterian Church and were living Christian lives.

A Korean Christian said to me one day: "I praise His name. When the missionaries came here they saved thousands of lives in their hospitals—not hundreds, but thousands."

ଓ ଓ ଓ

At a Korean Feast in Seoul

At a meal, the blessing is asked.

"This seems like such a fine thing to do," said Hong. "How did such a custom originate?"

"I never gave it a thought," said Dr. F. "I wonder if anyone present can tell the origin of grace at meals?"

Rev. S., the most recent missionary in Korea and fresh from Theology School, cleared his throat and hesitatingly volunteered, "I think I can give one explanation."

All the Koreans present, eager for information, watched him with increased admiration. "In the long ago, whole meals were prepared and offered on the altar of the gods. Later, only skin, bones, and the undesirable parts were offered. At a still later period, the food was only shown to the gods for approval. Perhaps there was a scarcity of food. Now, thousands of years later from the old pagan custom, we ask God to bless our food."

ଓ ଓ ଓ

Turning the corner we came upon a plump little Korean man with a pushcart that looked out of place among all the jiggies and rickshaws. When we heard the man call out his wares, we cocked our ears and listened again. To our surprise, what the man was actually saying was, "Li se Klim, li se Klim." "Come," said my companion. "Let's see what he has to offer." What he meant by "Klim," we never knew, but what he was serving was chipped ice in a little glass with a wooden spoon.

☙ ☙ ☙

In Hong Kong I saw a barefooted Chinese woman carrying a heavy load of bricks in two baskets swinging from a yoke on her shoulders. In addition to that load she had a baby strapped to her back. She was climbing a steep path up a hill where an English building was being constructed.

☙ ☙ ☙

Campaign against the three Ds: Dirt, Disease and the Devil.

☙ ☙ ☙

I went to a Japanese doctor to have my teeth cleaned. I told him I had a black deposit on my teeth ever since coming to Korea and asked the cause. He replied, "Tobacco." In that land both men and women smoke constantly.

☙ ☙ ☙

The Korean children have so little opportunity for education. Just now, a little ten-year old patient came hobbling in on his stick (we have no crutches for children) and said, "Please teach me." So I wrote "God" in Korean on a piece of paper for him. He is now working diligently, writing it over and over on the blackboard. This little patient came to the hospital six weeks ago with a tubercular hip and has been going around all this time with part of his body in a plaster cast.

☙ ☙ ☙

The Korean reasons that the tiger is the strongest animal in the country, and that the bone is the strongest part of the animal, so if you eat ground tiger bones you will be given strength. Logical isn't it?

☙ ☙ ☙

Korean Proverbs

(From *Life* magazine, July 10, 1950)
"Beware of the sword hidden behind a smile."
"The flower that blooms in the morning is withered by noon."
"A dead premier is worth less than a live dog."
"Pinch yourself and you will know the pain when another feels pinched."

೦౩   ೦౩   ೦౩

"No man ever worked his passage anywhere in a dead calm." -- John Neal

೦౩   ೦౩   ೦౩

Interesting experience in Cleveland hearing the famous Frenchman, Émile Coué, who advocated telling oneself, "Every day, in every way, I am getting better and better."

೦౩   ೦౩   ೦౩

Return to New York

As for Americans during this period, their thoughts were turned to many other things. They thought they were fighting a war to end all wars and deluded themselves into thinking they were making the world safe for democracy.

It was the era before jazz; a peaceful, contented age of waltzes and gracious living.

The three great captains of industry at this time were Thomas Edison, Henry Ford, and Harvey Firestone. The Barrymores ruled the American stage. Entertainment was provided by Fred Stone, Fritz Kreisler, and Oscar Hammerstein. Victor Herbert's "Naughty Marietta," "March of the Toy Soldiers," and "Kiss Me Again" were heard everywhere. The war songs "Tipperary" and "Over There" filled the air.

Decorum was passé. There was a slow death to conservatism. The shackles of convention were lifted. Sex was packed into everyday conversation. Sexy advertising and the era of the sex novels began to flourish.

Unfortunately, the experiment of prohibition resulted in speakeasies, bootleggers, and home brews. Cocktail parties flourished and women were becoming alcoholics. The moral fiber of the home began to break down, which would result in a great wave of juvenile delinquency. Far away in Korea, what we did not learn about America in our magazine reading, we caught up with when we returned home on furlough.

World War I Memories

"Over there, over there… And we won't come back till it's over, over there."

Marie Dressler - Douglass Fairbanks - Mary Pickford - Wilson - Teddy Roosevelt

Hinky Dinky Parlez Vous

Pack up your troubles in your old kit bag and smile, smile, smile

Kaiser - "All quiet on the western front"

Barbed wire fences and trenches

Wee, Wee, Marie (Oui, Oui, Marie)

Patriotic fever soared high

Winston Churchill

"Heaven, Hell, or Hoboken"

Allied break

Hindenburg line

Wilson's 14 points

Armistice – Nov. 11, 1918

50,000 never came home

The war to end all wars

Fog most terrifying to sailors

ଓ   ଓ   ଓ

When I first came to Korea, I wanted to teach all these ignorant people how to take care of themselves and their babies, and I thought my mission would not be fulfilled until I had taught them all how to care for their sick. I see differently now. My work as a missionary was to teach a few that I could gather about me, to influence and instruct them so that they could understand my message of cleanliness, health, and light; then let them in their turn teach their own people. At the end of my five years, I would be happy to have found two or three girls to share my vision of nursing.

"Life has taught me that no matter how tough the going may become at times, you do manage to get along somehow, by the grace of God."

Appendix II -- Notes on Nursing

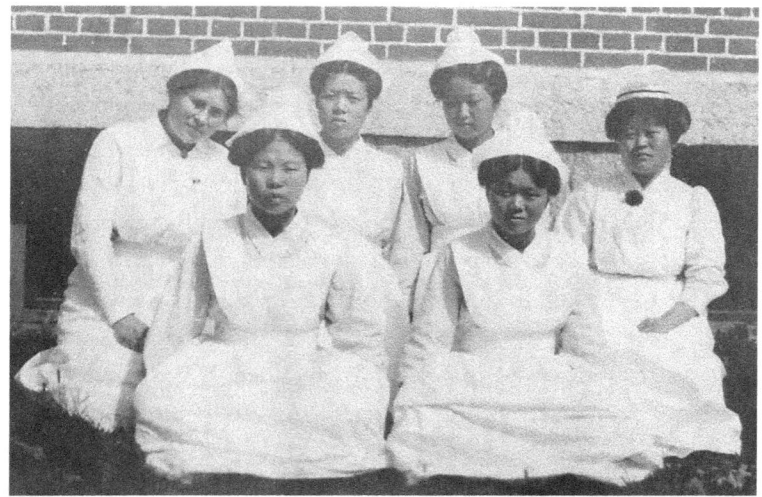

Delia, left, with Haeju nursing students

The following are miscellaneous notes on nursing experiences and thoughts about nursing as a profession.

Christian Careers Calling Nurses

It is now time to take a long view of the role of the missionary nurse. The present world-wide conflict[35] has brought mission work to a standstill in many lands. Nothing, good or bad, lasts forever, and this war will come to an end. When that time comes, Christian missions must be prepared to speed food, healing, and Christian comfort to a devastated world.

Relief must be given to masses of humanity currently engulfed in suffering: dislodged from their homes, threatened by disease, and made helpless by sickness and famine. A plea is now being made to prepare Christian nurses to meet this great need. Having a "divine calling" may be considered an old-fashioned expression today, but it best describes

---

35. The author refers to World War II.

the type of nurse needed for the mission field. The humanitarian ideal of service alone is not sufficient to qualify a nurse for mission work.

Following the last world war, two Red Cross nurses heard of the need for nurses in the Orient and decided to take advantage of an opportunity to gain valuable experience, as well as travel and adventure. When they arrived in the mission field, however, they could not adjust themselves. They just didn't fit, and were absolutely unable to begin working. It takes Christian grace to adapt oneself to the limited means of a mission hospital, cooperate with older missionaries, learn a new language, and in an inconspicuous way serve the people of another race.

Nurses responding to the call must feel deeply the inner urge to serve. They must be so fortified in Christian faith that they will make a place for themselves and be happy in the work. Besides the inner urge to serve suffering humanity, there are other qualifications that a missionary nurse must have, such as good health, a college education, and a graduate degree from an accredited school of nursing. Salary cannot be the primary consideration. At best, a nurse can hope to be provided with traveling expenses and support that is sufficient for a reasonably comfortable living. There is a pension plan based on years of service for missionaries. To justify the expense of travel, the first term of service is five years.

When this great world war is over, Christianity will bring healing to the nations. Young nurses must prepare to do their part. I have a message for Christian nurses who have a firm faith in God, and can step unafraid into greater fields of service: "the Master calleth for thee."

☙ ☙ ☙

"Developments in preventive medicine, particularly in the control of communicable diseases have been spectacular." The nursing field is changing. "The professional nurse must know the complex environmental and social factors that contribute to illness and that may in turn influence the degree of recovery and rehabilitation possible for the individual."

"For the want of the nail the shoe was lost, for the want of the shoe the horse was lost, for the want of the horse the battle was lost, for the want of the battle the kingdom was lost, all for the want of a nail."

"There are at least 25 national organizations devoted to child care."

"There are extremely interesting people hiding under the mantle of anonymity."

"Mental illness…may be due to functional disturbance due to boredom."

"Need recognition, novelty of experience, security and love."

"Was civilized and God-loving people, fighting to kill."

"I could not stand to hear them cursing God, for this was not God's work" (man-made war).

"They had no love of God, no fear of God," (they had no God at all).

"There 666 let up, we had to go on and on, take things as they come."

"Fight or die, fight or die, we must go on."

"More dead, more wounded, more dying."

"This was the Glory of War, `Bravo' shouted the Leaders (expendable) - but to the poor mutilated, shell-shocked men, it was Hell."—Private writings of Mrs. James Papalexis, 4110 Main Ave., Ashtabula, OH.

Personal Qualities of the Nurse

The competent nurse needs a sympathetic nature. She must be kind and thoughtful and without pity. She needs a sense of humor, a quality which serves well in every aspect of living. She needs tolerance, which must be based upon belief in the value of every life. She needs patience and tact—patients may become unruly and unreasonable at times. She needs flexibility—needless adherence to procedure achieves nothing and makes patients unhappy. She needs friendliness, warmth and genuine interest in people; patients are often lonely. She needs to manage patients without appearing to manage She needs teaching ability and physical energy. The nurse should be particularly observant of the emotional needs and reactions of patients. Signs of worry must be noted—worry and fear may often be allayed by careful explanation and reassurance, but also by letting the patient talk and express their fears. When listening to the patient, be aware of the need for assistance, for no patient is spared from the embarrassment of asking for help. Be aware of the need for privacy. Optimism is essential. Let patients do for themselves as much as possible—they need a sense of personal independence.

"Basic human needs: to love and be loved, secure companionship, recognition, and personal achievement."

"Society of Friends: people need 'somewhere to live, something to do, someone to care.'" "Need for belongingness. Economic security is less important than emotional security."

"We have an unusually high percentage of young people in our society, and even today half of our population is under 30 years of age."

All nurses know they have an opportunity given to few. At a time of sickness, they become part of the most sacred and intimate interactions of family life. In severe illness, all look to them. They are seen as pillars of strength. The nurse can do something that all the sympathy, love, and kisses of a devoted family cannot do. In their profession nurses are familiar with death. They learn about the intangible proximity of the other world when they see the spiritual radiance lighting up the face of one slipping quietly away.

Have you ever kept watch by the bedside of a feverish and delirious patient? Not so long ago that was almost all that could be done. Suddenly, the news flashed across the country that a wonder drug had been discovered. Subsequently, there appeared in rapid succession sulfa drugs and antibiotics such as penicillin, aureomycin, streptomycin and duracillin. Miracles occurred. We saw temperatures drop from as high as 105 to normal in 24 hours. Even the most dreaded diseases yielded swiftly to the new drugs. It was soon discovered they could be used as preventive measures; mastoid operations that used to be common are rarely seen now. Pneumonia responds so quickly to the wonder drugs that it can hardly be recognized today.

Nursing took me around the world and allowed me to serve people of all races, creeds, and colors. Lessons learned from nursing helped me care for and teach my children, as well as manage my home. Nursing was a profession I could fall back on if I was ever left on my own resources. I never realized the time would come.

Hospitals

Hospitals have changed today. They are no longer small, personal institutions with a nurse-superintendent in charge of the whole. Then, it was her hospital, her nurses, her doctors, and hours meant practically nothing. Personnel were truly working in the spirit of Florence Nightingale. Contrast that with the present situation. Hospitals have become large business enterprises run by administrators, functioning like large modern hotels—impersonal and departmentalized, with little or no emphasis on charity.

Radio

To all nurses: Your country needs you! Matchboxes - billboards - scholarships. A shortage of nurses is the greatest problem facing the profession today. Most nursing schools today require a high school diploma (with chemistry) and graduation from the upper half of the class, plus the ability to pass a pre-nursing examination.

Nursing: The career with a future for you! Check with the Director of Nursing at the nearest hospital that has a training school and gives a degree in nursing. It is an important decision to make if you want a really worthwhile career, a career that will allow you to spend your life helping other people—to see, walk, smile—even to live again.

Nursing

"Serious shortage of registered nurses today, so that nursing care is in the throes of an almost complete breakdown in many of our hospitals."

Unfortunate "experiences when they went to the hospital for a baby, to undergo an operation, or to be tested and treated."

Complaints are coming out of many hospitals. "Some told of never seeing a graduate nurse, or getting what little nursing they did receive from the hands of ill-trained practical nurses or virtually untrained volunteer aides."

"Ugly, shocking talk of the growing collapse of the greatest of nursing traditions—the nurse's first loyalty must be to her patient."

"The best nurses are aware that much is wrong with the profession. They're deeply concerned with restoring the fine tradition of service, which until recently has characterized their profession above all others."

There must be a trend back to the high ideals and principles of our profession. Nursing is a victim of the times; the whole belligerent attitude of labor today breaks down the inward satisfaction and joy in service. Nurses must remember that they are professional women, with professional dignity and standards to uphold.

Every man is worthy of his hire, but let's not allow the almighty dollar to motivate our objective for nursing. Rather, let service and a sympathetic love of our fellow man prompt us to choose nursing as our profession. In accomplishing that service let us always be motivated by the Golden Rule, to do unto others just as we would have others do unto us. When dignity is put back into labor, and labor does not exploit capital, then capital does not exploit labor.

There has been a shortage in the nursing and teaching occupations that has paralleled the emergence of women as a significant force in the political and industrial life of American culture.

Nurse!!!

"Learn to take care of others and you will always take care of yourself—study to be a nurse!" (Large billboard sign on a winding curve in the foothills of the Ozark Mountains, seen on California trip.)

My profession is a challenge and a great responsibility. It didn't take me long to find out how wonderful nursing is, how really satisfying it can be. I have often thought of my friends who were teachers, interior decorators, or musicians. In their professions they deal with pleasing or beautiful things, and they do not lose their identity as one of a group in starched uniforms. But I know I need not envy them, for deep down in my heart, I wouldn't change places with anyone. We nurses are familiar with birth, pain, death, miraculous recoveries, pains soothed, and discomforts eased. Girls who enjoy doing things for others, who are interested in worthwhile occupations, need to enter a profession like nursing. Recruits are urgently needed! Thousands of new professional nurses are needed today to meet the minimum health requirements of our own country. The experience will be invaluable; you will learn much about life. So many overwhelming things happen, yet one never ceases to marvel at the miracle of birth. I have lost all the sting and fear of death. It is not the worst thing that can happen to a person. Many times, I have seen it bring blessed relief. I have often been inspired by the radiance of people who have lived beautiful, consecrated lives, and then slipped quietly beyond the bend in the road.

"Every moment is precious, when a person's life hangs in the balance."

Skill, Courage, and Resourcefulness—Harry Emerson Fosdick of the Riverside Church, NY, tells the story of his father saying good-bye on the front steps of his house one morning: he said to his wife (Harry's mother), "Tell Harry that he can cut the grass today if he feels like it." Then after walking a few steps down the street, called back, "Tell Harry he better feel like it."

"If you don't get a task that you like, like the task you get."

Appendix III -- Obituary

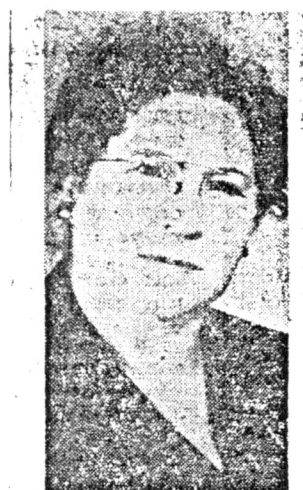

Mrs. William Lewis

Mrs. Delia May Lewis, 70 o: 6305 Edward Ave., died in General Hospital Friday morning Acute lukemia was given as the cause of death.

Born Dec. 3, 1888, in Plymouth she was the daughter of Eugene and Mary Mapes Battles. She attended City High School for two years and graduated from East High School in Cleveland. She attended Lake Erie College for two years and taught in Plymouth before entering Presbyterian Hospital Nurses Training School, Columbia University, New York City, where she graduated with honors in 1915.

A Red Cross nurse in World War I, she served eight months in Manchuria and Siberia. Following the war, she spent five years as a medical missionary in Korea, part of the time in Severance Hospital, Seoul. While there, she was instrumental in getting textbooks for nurses translated into the Korean language. She returned to this country by way of India and Europe completing a trip around the world.

She then went to Milford, Del., where she organized and opened the Milford Emergency Hospital and was its first superintendent. She later was supervisor of nurses in St. Luke's Hospital, Cleveland, returning to Ashtabula in 1924. During and since World War II, she has been engaged in private duty nursing.

Mrs Lewis has held the office of Regent of the Daughters of the American Revolution Regent of the Daughters of American Colonists, President of the Bunker Hill PTA, President of the Literary Society - Delphian Readers, President of the Ashtabula County Federation of Women's Clubs, President of the Missionary Society of First Methodist Church and Superintendent of the Junior Dept., Sunday School of the church. She was a member of the Zonta Club for many years representing the nursing profession.

Active in the Bible Club Movement, She had taught after-school classes for 10 years and had been a member of the Bible Club Council for 20 years, at one time serving as secretary.

She is survived by two children, Paul A. Lewis of Bellevue, Wash., and Mrs. Henry C. (Pamela) Goldman of Annapolis, Md. A sister, Mrs. O. L. Wright of Ashtabula two brothers, James Battles of Ashtabula and William Battles of Burt, N. Y., also survive as do four grandchildren, William A. and Valerie Ann Lewis of Bellevue and Mark William and Ned Lewis Goldman of Annapolis.

Her husband, William A. Lewis whom she married Aug. 1, 1924 in Cleveland, preceded her in death May 20, 1948.

Services are being held today at 3 .p. m. in Zaback Funeral Home with the Rev. W. E. Caskey Jr., of Lake Ave. Methodist Church officiating. Interment will be in Ridgeview Cemetery.

Appendix IV – Typescript of Letter from Miss Shields regarding Nursing Textbook

Jan. 5,1922.

Occidental Nurses Association,
Seoul, Korea.

        I wish to extend my heartiest greetings to the nurses of Korea. It was a pleasure and a help to me to be connected with the association while I was in Korea and I hope to be allowed to be your representative member in this country. Knowing the great amount of work that confronts you, and regretting that I am not there to share my part, I want to be ready from this side to do anything in my power to help with the work.

        The work of a nurse in a Mission Hospital is not easy. There was always so much to do and so few workers. We had to start in at our work before we could get a good knowledge of the language, and then with this handicap, we tried to train Korean nurses in our broken Korean. How we longed for a book in Korean that we could put into the hands of our nurses, so that they could read in their own language, the things we were trying to teach them. Literature and more literature for our Korean nurses was ever the crying need. During my whole five years on the mission field, I tried to contrive some way whereby we could have a nursing text book in Korean. It was a long struggle, with many difficulties to overcome, but the greatest difficulty came when, after we had gotten the book on the press we had to give up the whole proposition because we found that the translation of Maxwell & Pope, Bessie Kim had made was not clear in the Korean text.

        A text book in Korean we must have, and I thoroughly believe it will come about by the united efforts of all and surely the Occidental Nurses Association should rightfully handle the work.

        If the book is published in the name of the Occidental Nurses' Association with the title of "Maxwell and Pope Practical Nursing", printed in mixed script with the Unman at the side of the Chinese characters, I shall be glad to support the proposition in every way. I will turn over the permission I have received from the authors and publishers to translate and publish the book, also the cuts that are ready for the illustrations. And you can also use the money I have raised, several hundred yen, to carry on the work of translating and publishing. I shall want to know if more money is needed, for I shall probably be able to help more from the financial end of the work, than in any other way, because of being in this country.

        When the book is completed I wish three copies, two to present to each of the authors and one I should like for myself.

        Wishing you the greatest success in the work I remain,

                Sincerely yours,

Miss E.L.Shields R.N.
  Severance Hospital,
    Seoul, Korea.

www.ingramcontent.com/pod-product-compliance
Lightning Source LLC
Chambersburg PA
CBHW052027070526
44584CB00016B/1929